To Kathy

Health is wealth
nurture it

7/16/08

Optimum Health and Healing

Balancing Body, Mind, and Spirit

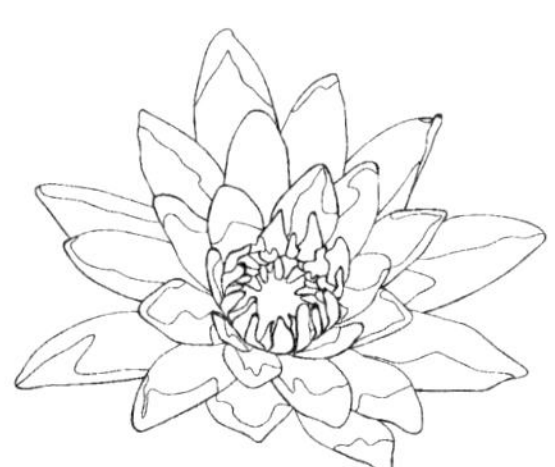

Dr. Mathew Maniampra, CMI

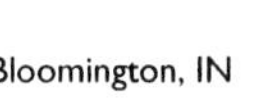

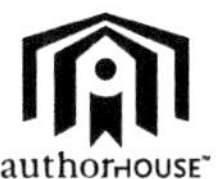

Milton Keynes, UK

AuthorHouse™
1663 Liberty Drive, Suite 200
Bloomington, IN 47403
www.authorhouse.com
Phone: 1-800-839-8640

AuthorHouse™ UK Ltd.
500 Avebury Boulevard
Central Milton Keynes, MK9 2BE
www.authorhouse.co.uk
Phone: 08001974150

First published by AuthorHouse 6/1/2006

ISBN: 1-4259-1797-6 (sc)

Library of Congress Control Number: 2006903064

Printed in the United States of America
Bloomington, Indiana

This book is printed on acid-free paper.

Optimum Health and Healing: Balancing Body, Mind, and Spirit

Dr. Mathew Maniampra, CMI – 1st Edition

www.optimumholistichealth.com

www.maniampra.com

Books By

DR. MATHEW MANIAMPRA, CMI

WHOLISTIC GROWTH: 100% LIFE

A SPIRITUAL VISION TO WHOLENESS

DR. MATHEW MANIAMPRA WEBSITES

www.optimumholistichealth.com

www.maniampra.com

DISCLAIMER

The information presented in this book is intended to help improve your overall well-being. It is not a substitute for appropriate medical care. I do not sell healthcare products or recommend any therapy or therapists. My task is to enlighten and awaken you with facts and information so that once informed, you can boldly move forward to create your own health. If you are facing a specific medical condition, be sure to discuss any lifestyle changes with your healthcare or medical provider.

IN APPRECIATION

I wish to express my sincere appreciation to all who dare to push the proverbial envelope on holistic health concepts, risking their own fame and name. I have many individuals to thank, especially my family and friends, who encouraged me and trusted me in their health crises. I am indebted to the many people who came to me in their stressful times of life regarding health and taught me many lessons.

Mathew Maniampra

To the

loving memory of my mother

now in Heaven

forever in my heart

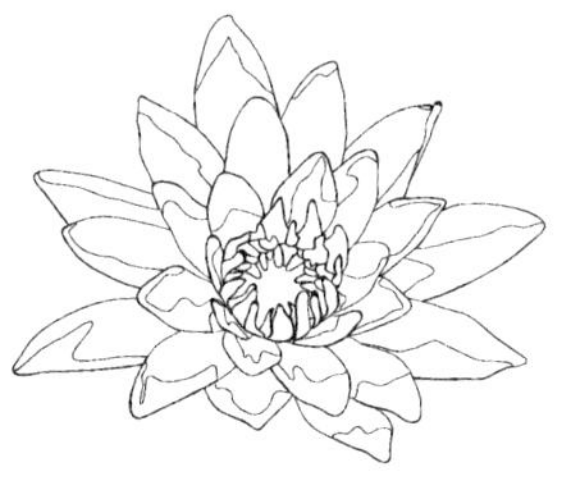

(1934 - 2003)

CONTENTS

Introduction

You may have recently visited a hospital or health practitioner. Perhaps, you may be taking some prescribed drugs or over-the-counter medicines. Irrespective of what the doctor said or diagnosed, you may have a gut feeling about your health. This gut feeling regarding your health is more important than the expert's opinion. So how do you rate your health? Excellent, good, fair or bad? The answer you give is a better indicator of your health and longevity than most medical indicators. Health, its meaning and value, is different for different people. Health and healing are not random phenomena. It is one's own creation to a great extent. Your personal involvement, beliefs, values, religiosity and worldview make enormous differences in the reality of health you experience.

In the past decade, we have witnessed powerful and rapid media-featuring health programs to promote the public health. The readily available and random piecemeal information streaming from various quarters of the medical community is confusing to many. We need a big picture, a complete know-how of the human organism. It is a machine and, yet, more than a machine. So much information is out there regarding the body, leaving aside other vital dimensions.

What is lacking is a total picture integrating the overlooked dimensions. When you buy any electronic item or machine, they all come with an operating manual. You open the box, pull out the manual and follow the step-by-step instructions for maximum performance.

No such comprehensive manual is out there to be applied in the case of humans for optimum health performance. No medical theory provides comprehensive understanding of what keeps people well or what makes them sick. An integrative medical theory and practice is still in its infancy.

My task, here, is to give a momentum to integrative medicine and the holistic health outlook dispelling common misunderstandings and misinformation.

Research in the field of medicine has revealed the flaw of the germ theory. Illness cannot be explained in terms of a germ theory or by some other external agent. This has left medicine with no adequate theory on the cause of diseases. We can rely on certain statistics on who will be at risk for a certain disease or under what circumstance one is likely to contract a disease. The field of medicine largely ignores the psycho-spiritual factors involved in the health crisis. Moreover, the medical profession is oriented toward directing and treating disease only after it reaches a point of crisis.[1]

Many people, even those who have the AIDS virus, never manifest symptoms. New studies increasingly show that emotions, attitudes, and beliefs are major factors in determining whether an individual exposed to the AIDS virus will develop the illness. A life that has minimum emotional disturbances develops a protective immune response and avoids having serious clinical illness. A sense of optimism and a positive outlook increases recovery after surgery. People who have a genuine religious commitment are seen maintaining better health and attain a speedier recovery in the wake of diseases. Their attitudes and outlook on life help them to keep at bay emotional disturbances that trigger a predisposition to illness. Religion as a rule promotes love, tolerance, compassion, forgiveness, hope and trust. Invoking these spiritual values to everyday life makes life more meaningful and purposeful. Meaning and purpose in life enhance the total quality of life and health.

Despite medical advances in health, we worry about health more than ever before. Where health and a long lifespan have been achieved, more fear and obsession in health is noted.[2] When you give one-sided attention to your body and health, you tend to assess the body negatively and make the worst assumptions. A preoccupation and concern with any organ might cause you to feel something strange about it. An individual who quiets the mind and learns to connect to the Transcendent by any religious practice will draw more of the qualities of the Transcendent they worship and trust. Connecting oneself to the Transcendent, the substratum of one's own being, will empower the person according to the overall purpose of life. We create the quality of our health in so many subtle ways. Our physical reality is actually created by an inner process.

> ***Our health is not created by external factors as medicine previously believed, but by many elements visible and invisible.***

People can deal with minor ailments and health problems which are a natural part of life and part of being human, provided they come to the awareness that the body is not only body – a physical entity

– but a spiritual embodiment with a purpose and meaning. Listening to the wisdom of the spirit, one can restore oneself to health or can comfortably cope with illness. Being attentive to one's body, mind, and listening to the spirit, we create health and healing and attain our destiny as is designed by the Higher Intelligence.

The holistic health view pays attention to the spiritual and emotional dimension of human life along with the physical problems. Informed alternative health practitioners can define the weak links in your body's structure and function and can direct you toward optimal personal care.[3] Holistic therapies do not in any sense make scientific medicine obsolete. It is still valid and a necessity in many medical problems. However, being wed to materialism, it lacks a comprehensive approach to build health and promote healing of people. Medical science's present perception of health is inadequate; it thinks every disease comes from the outside world. The holistic health view pays due attention to all the possible elements that can interact with our health system. There is no set therapy mode in the holistic approach to heal people.

There is no holistic technique to restore or build health; rather, it is a way of life and approach to health and healing incorporating different therapies, traditional and non-traditional. Sometimes traditional methods heal, other times they are helpless. Sometimes simple methods and techniques help. There is no single route to health that is equally applicable to all. In this book, therefore, you will come across various tips to health and healing drawn from different traditions and sources. In the end, health and healing is a mystery; still we struggle to fully comprehend it. We have only an occasional fleeting gaze into its true nature. By looking to materialistic medicine, we neither get glimpses into this mystery, nor can we deal with it properly. So, my attempt here is to give the reader a broader perspective in which to understand the phenomena of health and healing.

Disease is an imbalance and thereby an energy derangement in the organism moving from within to without. Any imbalance or disturbance felt by the entire organism is on all levels, but it is expressed sometimes on one level or another depending on the individuality of the patient. So, bodily symptoms are the end product of a process already started at some point in the past, which went unnoticed. In the pages to come, you will see that a religious commitment can be an important resource in maintaining physical and mental health. The mind quality one develops in life affects overall health and quality of life.

The best medicine is one that combines up-to-date medical technology, spiritual practices and mind training. Doctors who choose to ignore or are indifferent to the spiritual or mental concerns of the patient simply miss the opportunities to promote optimum health in their patients. Medical, mental, and spiritual professionals should learn to work together to provide the best possible care to the whole person. Though each profession needs to maintain some clear boundaries, blocking any kind of access to the medical, mental, or spiritual dimension by the other profession is not true professionalism. The walls between medicine and religion should come down. A rapidly growing number of medical schools have begun to incorporate spiritual disciplines in their curriculum.

By definition, faith transcends scientific method. Spirituality is not a thing to be tested and measured like other objects of science. However, the health benefits of spiritual commitment can be measured though we do not know exactly how it acts on the human being.

I have seen people desperately looking for healing. They are trained or conditioned to look in only one direction for help. I feel their pain and struggle could be lessened by having a different health understanding and by adopting sometimes a few simple techniques and lifestyle changes. We human beings are amazing creatures. There are hundreds of therapies that work and can yield results. A good number of therapies in vogue may not earn the scientific title. In each of you, there is something more than what simply scientific medicine can understand and verify. Miraculous healings happen everyday and everywhere that go against all scientific notions.[4]

It is my belief that this book will provide reason and rationale for a holistic health approach. For many, this will be a challenging journey to health. If this book stirs many questions in you regarding health or helps anyone to make a shift in the thinking about the nature of illness, health, and healing, I will have achieved my goal. Healing is a process that should begin from inside and to be complemented by external elements. Physical medicine would have been twice as powerful if it had paid due attention to the emotional and spiritual factors of human life. Isolating and treating humans solely as body, the mind and spirit have an imbalance and void in human life to be filled by disease of one sort or another in the long run. If your health is relatively good, this book will help you with more tips, information, and suggestions that you can translate into your life with a greater sense of well-being and happiness.

I

What Is Health?

Generally, health has been understood to be the absence of disease. The word *disease* comes from an old French word, meaning, "lack of ease." This lack of ease can originate from many sources, and need not be always related with the body. Health is more a sense of well-being of body, mind and spirit. You cannot create health with drugs, tonic, vitamins, exercise, nutritional information, etc. although these all may help. As long as our understanding of life and self is limited and narrow, we are handicapped in our ability to mobilize our inner resources to experience wholeness. Lacking a philosophy of health, scientific medicine tends to pay attention to the concrete manifestation of illness. A concept of non-material factors determining health and illness is totally lacking in orthodox medicine. Medical men and women who ignore the spiritual and emotional component of the human being are doing only a partial service to humanity. A philosophical understanding of life and the world is a prerequisite to understanding health in positive terms.

It is interesting to note that the words – *health and holiness* – come from the same root word "*wholeness.*" The connection of health to religiosity and religious practices is not something imposed at a later time. It arose so naturally from the early period of medicine. The word *medicine* comes from the Latin word "*medicina*" which gives us the words – *remedy, mediate, and measure.* The root suggests thoughtful action to establish order.[1] Medicine suggests actions to restore some aspect of wholeness implied by the word *health.* By definition, wholes are complete and perfect; they lack nothing. Moreover, in an ideal whole, components are not only all there; they are in an arrangement of harmonious integration and balance. In the strict sense, wholeness is the attribute of God, the creator. Man, the creature, becomes whole by integrating different components of his existence. Perfection and balance are traditional attributes of holiness. They also underlie the concept of health.

A long historical tradition connects religion, medicine, and health care. It was the religious establishments that built hospitals, provided medical training and licensed physicians to practice medicine.[2] Religion and medicine were closely linked until the advent of the scientific revolution. Indeed, the priest was the medicine man. Many cultures still regard the priest as a healer. By the end of the seventeenth century, there occurred a split between medicine and religion. The scientific profession of medicine nearly completely separated away from its religious beginnings. Over the past decades, the medical community has shown some interest in bringing down the wall that separated medicine and religion. The orthodox medical profession was compelled to do so by the emergence of research appearing in mainstream medical and public health journals reporting a connection between spirituality and health.

Health is wholesomeness; a flowing energy in harmony with the totality as each part relates and operates with the whole dynamically rebalancing, reconnecting and exchanging itself. The World Health Organization defined health as follows: "Health is a state of complete physical, mental, and social well-being and not merely the absence of disease or infirmity."

Science and medicine are rooted in the belief that scientific research can and will eventually discover the reason for all diseases that occur within and outside of us. Of course, science is able to provide some information relevant to disease, but its knowledge is insufficient, for science does not touch the inner realm of the human being. The journey to health involves a psychological and spiritual commitment along with addressing physiological problems.

The Mechanical and Materialistic View

People who see the human body as a machine treat it accordingly. When the body is considered a machine, the human being is viewed as nothing more than a warm-blooded automobile. Broken-down people may elect to go to surgery in order to be restored to health where they will be fixed by some experts in the field. Just as some mechanics only specialize in doing transmissions, some physicians only specialize in the heart; others specialize in the skin or the eye. Trouble comes when no broken parts can be found. Thorough exams sometimes reveal no underlying pathology, no broken parts and no sign of infection. In spite of the negative diagnosis, the patient feels he is disintegrating. Since humans are not simple machines, but a complex phenomenon, no single theory can explain away the human situation of illness, health, and healing. The mechanical view of medical science and its overdone specializations tend to focus on the bodily parts and disregard the individual. There is no single formula to "fix" a person lying in a hospital bed. You can take away the infection by antibiotics, replace or repair the broken-down parts, and can dull the pain with sedatives. Still, the person is not restored to the former state of his health, nor is he healed.

We human beings are body, mind, and spirit. How these dimensions of human existence are interconnected to act as one organism is little known. Nevertheless, an unbiased observer will feel an underlying unity among all the parts, which make a magnificent oneness in man. Despite our awareness of the complexity of the human organism, our tendency is to divide and conquer and to treat the human organism as separate entities. Thus, the body/soul dichotomy emerges as we observe it today. The body has an effect on the mind and the spirit; the mind affects the body and the spirit; the spirit affects the body and the mind. Scientific research in the last thirty years is replete with examples of mind/body interaction. Conventional medicine has inherent limitations because it is based on the concept of an isolated body/mind unit. Studies reveal that if a hospital room looks out on a garden or scenic spot, the healing of the patient is faster than if the room faces a brick wall. Because we do not fully understand how our bodies work, we think we have no power over health. Health is not gained by good luck nor is illness acquired often by fate.

Numerous researches have established a correspondent existence between the emotional and physical plane. Meditation increases circulation to the brain while producing relaxation to the muscular system, thereby lowering blood pressure. The state of fear creates palpitation of the heart, dry mouth, and perspiration of palms. Positive emotions of love and compassion can create positive effects in the body.

Every stimulus, every thought, every emotion, has a corresponding effect to some degree on all levels of the body simultaneously and instantaneously.

A number of illnesses are psychosomatic – no physical reason for them. When we say something is psychosomatic, we do not mean there is lack of pain and suffering. Pain, suffering and tissue damage are real. One may feel all the symptoms of real sickness; the only difference is that its genesis is from the mind and not from the body.

All illness affects mind and body. The body is the physical part of our existence. The mind is the non-physical, spiritual aspect of our being. They work together, they interact, they complement, and interpenetrate each other. You have no existence without the mind, and you have no existence without the body. The mind is real but it cannot be measured and detected like physical organs. All our human illnesses are colored or shaped by the characteristic of the mind of the person who owns it. In a number of cases, symptoms of illnesses are caused by the mind more than any other agents. It is not the bacteria and viruses that first appear. They are like scavengers. They reach the spot where your vitality is weakened by mental and spiritual stress.

Medical science in the last few decades has agreed that the mind has a role in making people sick or well. Mostly, this finding remains in the theoretical realm. Only when extreme distortions of mental disorders occur, any serious thought is given to it. And whenever there is serious distortion in the functioning of the mind, it is treated in isolation. Psychiatry deals with the mind that is reduced to a neuro-chemistry and biological process. Here also the individual is left out. Every human life incorporates physical, mental, emotional and spiritual components. Many systems or philosophies of healing operate under the assumption that man is a composite organism. Healing occurs when giving a balanced thought to all these elements that make us human.

Western science is based on the belief that consciousness arises from the matter, awareness being a product of the physical process occurring in the nervous system and brain. In the perspective of Eastern philosophy, consciousness shapes the physical world and our experience of it. Our dread of pain, fear of disease, and experience of pleasure all depend on the state of our consciousness. The mind and consciousness are tools the spiritual self possesses for its self-realization. Therefore, what was perceived by an unenlightened mind as mere weakness or powerlessness can be perceived as messages for change and transformation.

Man being essentially spiritual, a spiritual outlook can set off healing forces from within.

Medicine denied consciousness as a determinant of health and healing that held sway until recently. The Newtonian view of matter and energy as quantities independent of the mind led to this attitude. Rene Descartes (1596-1650) pioneered the movement of strict separation of mind and matter. Thereupon, everything that affects the body was explained in terms of mechanics. For a long time, the model of the universe was an orderly mechanism that goes lawfully about its business unaffected by any mind behind it.

Recent research in the field of body, mind, and spirit challenge the traditional assumptions about what it means to be human, how we become sick, and how we attain health. The body-mind approach – or psychosomatic medicine – is a step in the right direction. But it has not gone far enough. There is something more to attaining health than just having good genes and cells in our body. A sound mind and right attitude help to a great extent to attain health. Besides medicine, so many other elements sometimes can take you a long way in the process of healing. There is something more in the human body that cannot be accounted for even by the best psychosocial theories or the principles of behavioral medicine.

The assumption – body as machine – still holds sway in most medical specialties. This is evidenced by the continued attraction of costly, high-tech diagnostic, and therapeutic procedures.[3] The new health model will not be grounded principally on genetics and molecular biology; instead it will be founded on an integrated body, mind, and spirit perspective. Present day orthodox or conventional medicine is built on the biomedical model that does not even partially answer the health problems.

Primacy of the Spirit

I recently was called by one of my friend's family and told the bad news that came after visiting the doctor's office. Richard was diagnosed with prostate cancer; and he was in great distress. He was fifty-five years old. He feared he would not live long. He said, "I am only fifty-five; I haven't lived my life fully." He had a feeling that this situation was unfair. I conversed with him for almost an hour. He was not sure whether he should go for chemotherapy along with its painful results, or go for radiation therapy. Instead of steering him to a particular healing modality of chemotherapy or natural healing methods, I tried to connect him with his inner realm. I motivated him to search his own inner spirit and connect himself to his inner self before rushing to any treatment models. When we finished, he was in a state of acceptance and less nervous. After calming him, I encouraged him to pray with me. Though he was religious, at this point I found he needed some support to turn to in his inner realm.

Man is essentially a spiritual being. So, when he connects himself with his spiritual essence, it is felt in every aspect of his life even in his every cell. Prayer and faith involves opening our hearts and communicating in some way or other with a greater presence and power. This sense of being associated with a higher concerned power is simply enough to calm down and soothe the nerves.

Generally, people rush to doctors and treatments to heal themselves. They surrender to the doctor and medicine before they are able to pull themselves together by taking sufficient time. All healing comes from within and from the body's own ability to heal itself. So, the first thing shall be to look in and connect with one's own resources. Before we go outside seeking remedies, we should go first inside of ourselves. If we do the first thing first, we will be in a better position to get the maximum benefit from other sources. First, make a spiritual connection to your inner self via your faith and prayer. Fostering the spirit within you is your first line of defense against illness and the most important tool in healing. A spiritual outlook can set off healing forces from within. It shall be the first step.

The spirit is integrally and intimately connected with the body and the mind. We know our body through our five senses. Using our senses and our reason, we explore the world. We cannot know the spirit in the same way we know the world and the body, for the former is related but not confined to it. It is more elemental and basic than what we can obtain through our five senses, nervous system, and the brain. Aldous Huxley, English poet and essayist, remarked: "The brain, nervous system, and sense organs are given to us to narrow the vast range of experience of which we are capable and to focus our attention in order to survive."[4] All religions hold the view that we have other ways of achieving this; they are found in meditation and the mystical experience.

Morton Kelsey, in his book *Christopsychology,* opined that we are immersed in a spiritual world, and when we do not deal with its contents as consciously as possible, these contents deal with us.[5] When we are completely cutoff from the spiritual realities, which have a direct bearing on our lives, the result is that we are plagued by numerous anxieties, phobias, irrational compulsions, addictions, fears, feelings of helplessness, despair, and meaninglessness of life. These experiences emerge into the body in the form of physical problems and illnesses. Kelsey reminds his readers that the only thing more dangerous than dealing with the spiritual reality is not dealing with it. Karl Jung came to the same conclusion in the 1920's that most neuroses in people over thirty-five were the result of being cut off from the reality of which all the great religions speak.

The mechanical worldview maintained that we can understand the function of every cell, organ, and human system, and can replace them with new ones. Within the strictures of the mechanical worldview, the human being is a physical structure with chemical and physical characteristics that can be manipulated, including the mind, emotions and spirit, with no input from the invisible realm. In contrast to the mechanical worldview of traditional medicine, holistic therapies and medicines have acknowledged the role of the human spirit in health and healing. Health, illness, and healing are related concepts. We cannot deal with one without touching the other. Each person creates consciously or unconsciously the creation of his own reality, including the reality of his health. The tools that create our health and illness are our attitudes, emotions, and belief patterns as well as the awareness of our own spiritual selves.

Like Jung, Robert Assagioli observed that in the ideal human development there is a turning to the spiritual and transcendent during a mid-life transition.[6] Contemporary psychologists and thinkers consider the vocation of a human being to be the attainment of wholeness by finding the unity of the self. Unlike Freud, most psychologists today acknowledge the primacy of the human spirit in the human existence.

Today, most people know the mind affects the body, but how the spirit affects the body and mind may be new to many. (I refer here to the spirit to denote the religious dimension of the human organism.) Most illnesses are the outward expressions of the crisis of the spirit. Our human spirit needs attention and care. To live healthily, one needs to make a balance between the spiritual, mental, and physical values of life. When a person continuously lives in a material realm devoid of any spiritual values, an imbalance is created so much so that every cell of the organism wants to correct it and sends internal messages or signals accordingly. Sometimes it will take the form of localized symptoms, and if not heeded, it would then shake-up or affect the whole system.

Consciousness is whispering its wisdom to us sometimes through bodily and mental problems. Our body and mind sound differently but both are governed by an intelligent self or consciousness. This intelligence can express itself in the form of an energy pattern. Consciousness is energy in its subtle and finest form. Consciousness naturally makes its impact first on the mental and spiritual realm, for they are of the same immaterial nature.

It seems that when the spirit is touched or awakened, healing is miraculous and quick. Since this is an interior realm, which is not observable or quantifiable, the scientific world is at a loss to understand this phenomenon.[7] The human spirit is integrally connected with the physical organism in a single integrated totality. An ancient Sumari text puts it rightly: "Honor your body, which is your representative in the universe. Its magnificence is no accident. It is the framework through which your works must come. The flesh and spirit are two phases of your actuality in time and space. Who ignores one, falls apart in shambles."

Nonetheless, one thing is obvious; there is an interconnection and interaction between body, mind, and spirit. Therefore, when physicians become technicians of the body, psychologists technicians of the mind, and zealous clergy keepers of the soul, the result naturally will be the missing of the human person. What and where influence begins and ends is sometimes difficult to locate in the highly complex phenomenon of human beings. So, we need to be open to all different possibilities.

> ***Choosing health is not simple, for no one factor determines health. It is the result of countless interrelationships in the web of life, where everything relates to everything else.***

When scientific medicine rejects other therapies and techniques because they do not conform to the strict scientific standards, it is the rejection of the dignity of the human being, which has a triune nature and magnificent oneness. Because of this triune and complex nature of the human being, one has to acknowledge that there is an ever-present danger of overlooking one dimension against the other. Sometimes we tend to spiritualize psychological realities and psychologize spiritual realities; at other times, we simply interpret everything as a mere physiological process.

Most religious traditions envision the body as the lowest part – the most visible and tangible part. The visible and tangible is not the paramount portion of the human organism. It is just a beginning; it is a gate to enter the center. The body is throbbing with a presence that is invisible. The mind can shape the flow of energy that in turn determines what happens on the physical level. Although the mind plays an important role, it is not the ultimate causal force in creating health and illness. There is something beyond the limited mind that shapes it.

The connection between body, mind, and spirit means that a problem originating in one part may affect the other and, thereby, upset the whole balance of the organism. The way our mind perceives the reality may affect the whole function of the body. Inadequate nutrition and chemical imbalances may cause physiological depression in human beings. The human spirit, when starved, shows itself in different forms such as meaninglessness, boredom, loneliness, lack of contentment, inability to forgive, feelings of depression and restlessness. All these factors in turn affect the immune system, functioning and health. Caroline Myss and Norman Shealy boldly state, "Time has come to assert one primal fact: the human spirit is real. Beyond the chemical, psychological, and physiological study of the disease, there comes a point, as we search for the cause of illness, when we are led to the core of a person's spirit."[8]

No Perfect Health

In this planet, everything exists in relation to the other, a balance of opposite forces. The possibility of pain refers to the existence of pleasure. Philosopher Alan Watts has expressed it, "Because human consciousness must involve both pleasure and pain, to strive for pleasure to the exclusion of pain is, in effect, to strive for loss of consciousness. Light is white only because it contains a mixture of many different colors and hues other than white." Health, like light, is also a mixture. Human experience is made possible only through contrasts. Health, like light, cannot be pure; it must contain an opposite balancing element, namely, illnesses for the experience of health.[9] So, perfect health will remain an illusion.

Illness and health are not pure independent states. One is the necessary other half that completes the whole. As they are interrelated and contribute to make the whole, methods of science cannot analyze and understand them fully. They are rooted in the mystery of being. The mystery of being is not the realm of science but philosophy. Therefore, medical science can never fully comprehend health and sickness. Wholeness results from accepting the dark aspects, the shadows of our being, and transcending them.

The yin-yang symbol of Taoism graphically expresses the truth of perfection attained by an interaction of complementary opposites. The yin-yang symbol and philosophy behind it gave rise to the theory and method of Chinese medicine.[10] The medical emblem "Caduceus Wand" represents two snakes spitting at each other. At the top of the wand are light and dark, good and evil, yin and yang. More interesting, the snakes that twine around the wand are not dead or frozen; they are in dynamic action. Healing energy and power flow freely when the complementary opposites of existence are interwoven into a perfect pattern. The medical emblem signifies this vital truth. Sadly, this rich and powerful concept has been overlooked by orthodox medicine for a long time.

People can achieve a higher health experience by heightened awareness. They experience illness as a natural part of life. If the disease disappears, they are grateful; if not, they also have reasons for gratitude. A sense of gratitude always stirs up a sense of well-being meaning in life despite illness. People of higher health come to the awareness and realization that physical illness, no matter how painful or grotesque, is of secondary importance in the total scheme of existence. This is the awareness that one's authentic self is completely impervious to the ravages of any physical ailment. The disease may regress or disappear when this awareness is drawn for reasons we do not fully understand.[11]

Perhaps, when people find meaning and purpose in life that becomes a source of strength and energy, it unleashes some healing powers from within.

Human Uniqueness

The nature of the human being as such, oftentimes health and healing assume a dimension that defies human logic and understanding. Health is wholeness, the achievement of balance in the organism with nothing left out and everything in just the right order.

Certain personality features help people to be adaptive in recovery. The better problem solvers, people who directly confront problems, have better recoveries. As individuals are unique, what heals them is unique, too. What is perceived perfectly good to heal one person may not achieve the same result in another.

The field of health does not always follow the cause and effect pattern of physical science. There are people who violate every rule of health; still they rarely get sick. Heavy smokers do not always develop lung cancer. Likewise, alcoholics do not always develop cirrhosis. A high-fat diet need not lead to atherosclerosis and heart attack. Not all promiscuous people contract AIDS or sexually transmitted diseases. Without any medical work, sometimes a lump disappears. One might say it is their luck, genes, heredity, stars, etc. What makes health and what makes healing is sometimes beyond our rationale.

Scientific medicine does not respect the invisible and mysterious. Because our spirit is transcendent in its nature, our health and healing always have an element of a transcendental quality, which prevents us from forming clear-cut principles and laws governing the healing phenomenon. All different kinds of healing and healing modalities only highlight how complex our human nature is and often beyond our comprehension. Healing of any kind involves an element of mystery, too. This will become more obvious as we proceed to the next chapters.

2

Holistic Perspective of Health

I have seen many patients taking a pill for blood pressure, another for diabetes, yet another for cholesterol, and a different one for arthritis. As time goes on, they will make more regular visits to the hospitals and will take more doses with greater frequencies. The journey to health involves not regular visits for a checkup, but addressing nutritional deficiencies, cleaning up the toxins from the system, watching stress levels, eating well, exercising, keeping the right environment, as well as attending to one's mental and spiritual needs.

Ancient and New

A holistic health approach was the order of the most ancient civilizations. In the holistic health view, the body, mind, emotions and energy are related to the realm of the spirit. The body is not a mere body. It is a vehicle to achieve one's ultimate end. This view of the ancient's was totally disregarded with the emergence of the scientific era of medicine. It is again rediscovered in the past decade beginning from the 1970's. It is in Cicero's works that we come across the first holistic view. He says, "A careful prescriber, before he attempts to administer a remedy to a patient, must investigate not only the malady of the person he wishes to cure, but also his habits when in health, and his physical condition." The picture of an individual's normal state of wellness is a prerequisite for the right kind of treatment. So, it is important to know what kind of person has the sickness. This is equally as important as who has the illness.

All disease results from a combination of genetic and environmental factors. Disease is the result of an imbalance in the system, not the cause of it. Symptoms are only a message that there is an imbalance. If the therapy orients to treat only at the physiological or symptomatic level, we are not doing a real service to the patient. The individual may receive symptomatic relief temporarily, but a real sense of well-being and health will ever be missing which, in turn, leads to stress and further diseases.

Properly speaking, there exists no holistic medicine. It is an informal collection of practices and attitudes, not a defined system of treatment. The term *holistic* is loaded with a lot of positive things for those who like it and negative for those who have a different philosophy and/or values. The holistic medical movement began in the 1970's as a reaction to the excesses and deficiencies of conventional medicine. It is more a health movement than treating disease. Holistic medicine as the term implies takes into consideration the whole person and his individuality. A complete picture of the patient is needed to individualize the treatment.

Reductionism

Science has a tendency to narrow down its focus to the phenomenon it observes. It likes to break down things into minute particles and atoms that it can confidently handle and exercise some level of control. Natural objects and things studied through this reduction method have their advantages. But, the advantage is limited when focusing on humans. Human understanding is limited and determined by its conceptual modes. Our understanding of any object is limited proportionately to the images we conjure up on a field we want to perceive.

If we cannot envision images and pictures in the first place, our understanding is almost at zero level. In the medical field, where reductionism has been the rule, the whole image of health is lacking. The advent of the hologram has offered a new template for conceptualizing how parts of a living system reflect the whole.[1] The holographic metaphor implies that each piece contains the essence of the whole. Each cell in the body, or tissue, or organ, embodies somehow the quality of the whole and has a tendency to manifest the whole. The holistic view envisions the individual system as part of a greater encompassing natural order. This perspective gives a new appreciation of the ancient traditions of diagnosis. Every tissue and organ can give certain information about the functioning of the whole. So, we can look at the face of the person, palms, eyes, skin, etc., and all can bring up some impression to make a whole image. The narrow data emerging from laboratory tests and cursory examinations appear to be like looking at an object from one specific angle. A holistic diagnosis brings information and impressions from a different spectrum and puts it together intuitively. Intuitive faculties are likely to play a major role in every diagnosis even in the high-tech tests when doctors look at X-rays, CAT and MRI scans, etc. And as we know, no two doctors interpret the results in the same fashion. Palmistry, long dismissed as superstition, takes on an intriguing new potential when we begin to think in holographic terms.

No Single Cause

Conventional medicine lacks a unified concept of health and healing. It considers disease as an external attack, more than a failure of normal homeostasis, (a relatively constant state with the body, naturallly maintained). There is a widely held misconception that illnesses are caused by germs, viruses, and bacteria from the outside. The enemy is always out there in this medical model. As the result of this misconception, the interior realm of the human person and the role of consciousness is underestimated or overlooked. From the holistic perspective, disease is generally considered the integrated result of all cosmic, environmental, chemical, electrical, mental, physical, emotional attitudes and spiritual stress. In fact, there is no single cause. As there is no single cause, there is no single remedy. Since the individual health is the sum total of all the above-mentioned elements, emphasis shall be on keeping the homeostasis and balance rather than redressing a problem element.

A given cause may produce no illness or a conceivable illness, depending upon the constitution of the person, which is the result of genes, habits, conditioning, etc. Studies show that most lung cancers are the result of smoking. Still the question remains, why do all smokers not contract lung cancer? Why do all alcoholics not die of cirrhosis? You must have noticed some people survive unbelievably serious injuries with no apparent damage, while some others die or have various types and degrees of dysfunction from minor injuries. Johns Hopkins Medical School conducted studies on this question and found a correlation with personality types.[2] Relative specific personality types predispose one to high blood pressure, tuberculosis, heart attack or even cancer. These traits are present twenty or thirty years before the onset of the disease. Eric Berne, the great psychiatrist in *Games People Play,* demonstrates that we develop a script at the early age of life, and play it back later.[3] It seems that the majority of individuals decides at an early stage of life both the age and course of death. If we choose the course of death and illness, it must be possible to choose health also. We can choose our life scripts. In the healing works and approach, all these are to be analyzed and should help people to make new choices or to rewrite the script in a healthier way.

Smoking is not the only cause of lung cancer. Physical factors seem to provide only one level of influence in people's lives. The missing factors are related to the subjective life of the individual and the immeasurable areas of emotions, attitudes, and spiritual stress. Oftentimes, the spiritual stress is the root of many illnesses. The root of spiritual stress is the fear of the loss of life, health, money, love or values. These fears lead to anger, guilt, depression, and frustration. Spiritual stress originates from lack of true perspective and understanding about the nature of life and its goal and meaning.

Rick Warren in his remarkable book *The Purpose Driven Life* states, "Everyone's life is driven by something."[4] Many people are driven by guilt, others by resentment and anger; still others by greed or fame; a few others by the need for approval and success. How much you are driven and in what fashion you are driven causes stress and is to be explored for a healthy life. Your spiritual attitudes and values determine the nature of the stress you undergo. Sensing our spiritual identity, that is immutable and imperishable, and our unity and oneness with all others will produce the needed attitude to handle life in a healthy fashion.

Health begins from the holistic perspective, with a conscious determination to grow optimally in expressing the spiritual goals. Healing of the spirit and, thereby, the emotions are essential for healing of physical diseases. Drugs and surgery are giant bandages in acute situations to help patients, until they can develop an inner strength to enter consciously into their spiritual selves and transform themselves.[5]

It is the experience of holistic healers that physical interventions coupled with psycho-spiritually oriented ones make positive measurable differences in health and wellness. Because we are primarily spiritual beings in our core, spiritual stress can cause a lot more stress in our lives than we can imagine. Without feeling, touching, and sensing the core of our being, what one can have and receive is cosmetic health only – never true health and quality of life. We humans are trained to conceive a perfect body and health.

Contemporary psychologists and thinkers consider the vocation of the being to be the attainment of wholeness by finding the unity of self with the Universal Self. When people are out of touch with the inner dimension of life, there is a chance that they are plagued by numerous anxieties, phobias, irrational compulsions, and addictions.[6] It is the perfect spirit that one needs for a healthy body, not vice versa. The cause of illness and healing factors are more psychic and spiritual than physical. This is a bit in contrast to the traditional medical notion that it is the physical world that contains the forces that exert the strongest influence on the body.

Why do people develop illness? When a diagnosis is received, everybody tends to ask the question: "Why did this happen to me?" In the case of a few, it is explainable if they have abused their bodies by smoking, drinking, or exposing themselves to a hazardous environment. For the vast majority, there is no answer to the question "Why?" People at one time turned to religion for answers. Indeed, throughout history religion, spirituality, and the practice of medicine have been intertwined. As a result, many religions took it upon themselves as a sacred duty for the caring of the sick. Many of the world's leading medical institutions have religious and spiritual roots. When people consult physicians to determine the nature of their disease, they also are asking some questions in their internal forum. Why is this happening at this moment in my life? How does it fit into the overall purpose and meaning of life? Features of spirituality include the quest for meaning and purpose, transcendence, and connectedness. Religion and spirituality are among the most important cultural factors that give structure and meaning to human values, behaviors and experiences.

Curing and Healing

Physicians see disease as the malfunctioning of the physiological or psychological processes. Health is seen as a static state and disease is a departure from this state. Curing is returning to the optimum static state. Disease is that malfunctioning level in your system caused by internal or external stimuli. Illness, on the other hand, is the individual's experience of the disease that is unique. To put it in a different way, disease is something an organ or a system has; illness is something an individual has. This distinction impacts the treatment and reveals the contrast between curing and healing.

Medicine, in general, has amassed a great deal of information concerning human beings from anatomy, pathology, biophysics, biochemistry, psychiatry, and so on. If the heart is affected, we treat the heart; if the liver is affected, we treat the liver. Cure is confined to treating symptoms or reactions. 'Cured' means treated with drugs or surgery until the symptom disappears. Authentic healing is more comprehensive. It touches upon the physical, psychological and spiritual factors. Healing must be looked at in a much broader sense than just changes in the body and symptom relief. Whether or not a desired cure takes place, healing is available to all. A healed person will be the owner of an enriched life, with a sense of fulfillment, inner freedom, creativity and vitality. These are not generally related to the state of simple physical health. In other words, healing will bring about a qualitative life rather than a quantitative life.

In medical science, the biochemistry of a molecule was more valued than the human person. Medical science failed to develop a system of reference that applies to the whole person and not just the organs and tissues. It is Dr. George Engel in the 1950's who established the "bio-psychosocial" model as a way of looking at treating all aspects of the patients – their psychological milieus as well as the biological perturbations accompanying the disease of mind and body. Eventually, the physician's interest shall change from prescribing the right medications to getting the patient off the medications altogether. Thomas Edison prophetically envisioned it when he remarked, "The doctors of the future will give no medicine but will interest his patients in the care of the human frame – and in the cause and prevention of disease."

In traditional curing, what counts is the blood pressure, the fractured bone, the migraine, etc. The person in whom the malady resides is irrelevant. Sometimes curing is impossible but healing is the only solution. In order to be healed, a different set of attitudes, beliefs and values is needed. Curing and healing are not synonymous. The medical community has begun to understand lately that a cure is impossible in a given situation, but healing is possible.

Individuals vary in their ability to withstand pain. Socio-economic and cultural factors play a role in the experience of pain. Several studies state that beliefs formed in socialization contribute to our threshold for pain. Religious values, upbringing, and heritage decide how you are going to put up with your pain. Our communities, governments, organizations, and above all, the media, tell us what to fear and what to avoid. We are told to avoid pain at any rate. Numerous ads appear everyday to relieve pain. They give the impression of a painless life with 100% life enjoyment. The more we see such a pain-free life shown to us by the powerful media, the more we tend to expect it. Then, when one brushes with reality, the more it hurts. Chronic diseases are on the rise. More and more people are about to suffer from chronic problems. The promise of quick fixes and miracle cures raises the bar of expectation high, so that eventually many suffer from depression. Rather than an unrealistic expectation of cure, the maximum comfort and mobility can be the maxim so that the body may assimilate such images and ideas and wire itself to cope with the inevitable in a graceful way.

No Guarantees

Health being the primary wealth and tool for success and happiness, it is natural for humans to look for all kinds of therapeutic methods to be healed. There is no guarantee that medical technology, therapeutic methods, religious commitment, natural lifestyle, etc. can restore health. As we have seen earlier, many factors interact to keep a dynamic equilibrium in humans. No surgeon can guarantee a safe recovery. When a skillful surgeon performs heart surgery or a kidney transplant, the chances are good that you will survive and experience few, if any, complications. But even under the best of circumstances, some patients experience complications and may die. It cannot be attributed to the impotency of the doctor or medical technology. We cannot fully decipher why some people develop complications, when in a given situation it should not have occurred. There seems to be a mysterious and transcendent factor in human health and healing. Not all who pray for healing are healed, even if it is offered by the holiest person with an ardent faith. Neither religious commitment nor medical treatment, or both together, can offer a guarantee for the recovery. Medical science operates on probabilities, not certainties. It is a myth that all can be treated and restored to health.

A cure is impossible in a given situation, but healing is possible.

Religious commitment is a critical factor in the healing process, but no one can force God to act. No one can manipulate God or control God's power of healing. You cannot predict when God's grace reaches you or not. We operate on probable outcomes. If we are to treat the whole person, we must consider the patient as a spiritual being as well as a biological, psychological, and social being. Religion and medicine are twin traditions of healing. To reconnect the two traditions of faith and medicine, doctors will need to learn a great deal about how exactly religiosity helps people stay healthier, recover from illness, live longer, and experience greater satisfaction and will need to be willing to incorporate a respect and sensitivity to spiritual values and practices in clinical care.[7] Recently, the *American Psychiatric Association* has developed guidelines to promote the inclusion of spirituality in psychiatric residency training. This development represents a major revolution in the field of psychiatry whose founding father, Sigmund Freud, denounced religion as universal neurosis.

The Meaning of Illness

At a glance, illness and its subsequent suffering have no meaning and purpose. One may feel it is simply there to make life miserable. The fragmented view of materialistic medicine does not present any meaning and purpose to your suffering. One has to find it from an existential and spiritual way. Anyone who receives a diagnosis of serious illness automatically tells oneself, 'I want to live.' This is more a reaction to fear than the will to live. The will to heal is a far greater commitment to the healing process. It is the capacity to enter into a journey of transformation, exteriorly and interiorly. Healing is healing only when it touches the inner core of the individual and helps for a transformational process toward wholeness. The annals of medicine are full of case histories of people who should have lived, but died because of their weakened will or spirit. Harnessing the sick person's will to live is central to healing.

The will to heal involves the preparedness to take up an inner journey, which entails some sort of suffering. People of higher health come to the awareness and realization that physical illness, no matter how painful and grotesque, is at some level of secondary importance in the total scheme of existence.

Suffering is part of the healing process. This may sound weird to many. Remember, that which hurts teaches and prompts us to look in and out to see what is wrong. It challenges us to make strong decisions. Suffering teaches us about our dark sides, our inner strengths, and our capacity to rise beyond our previous limitations. It can be a shedding process, a letting go of the various parts of ourselves that interfere with the development of our innerselves.[8] It relates us to a higher and spiritual purpose of life. It would seem that our tendency to suffer would greatly be diminished if we were able to recognize the spiritual wisdom inherent in the natural continually changing process of our lives.

Viktor Frankl made it known to the world that suffering can be a means of self-realization depending on the attitude one takes. This concept is wonderfully exemplified in his work, *Man's Search for Meaning.*[9] Self-realization through meaning is the highest form of achievement according to Frankl. When we have meaning, we have reason to live and thereby affirm existence even under the worst conditions or situations. When life is found with meaning and affirmed, a sense of well-being and healing comes to us. A sense of wholeness is experienced in spite of pain and suffering.

Our ego is the receptacle of our fears, needs, and insecurities. In our spiritual self, we do not have any insecurities and fears. Ego keeps drawing attention to itself because we have conditioned it to do so. In the Freudian personality theory, ego is required. Without developing a strong ego, a healthy personality is impossible. Ego wants the world to swirl around it. It makes us believe that it is the center of our being and the world itself. It rebels against any change that is not immediately satisfying and pleasurable. Ego, therefore, is not willing to take any pain to find out the meaning of illness, nor does it want healing if it goes against immediate gratification. Healing and self-realization come when one is able to go beyond the personal identity. Ego is a liability in healing because of its controlling needs and insatiability. Upon realizing the nature of this ego, one may free oneself from its clutches; if not, growth and healing may not occur. Because ego keeps drawing attention to itself, the spiritual self is overlooked or forgotten. It is the part of us that is connected to the universal consciousness and to all of life. So long as the ego has its grip on us, the spiritual part is not able to guide us towards our destiny. It is this spiritual self that holds the power to heal. This spiritual self is referred to in different disciplines with varying terminologies such as Universal Energy, Vital Force, Higher Consciousness, etc.

Renouncing the individual ego identity is a prerequisite for healing, transformation and self-realization. For many, illness is chronic, even life-long. The loss of limbs, disfigurement, and/or permanent disabilities is sometimes irreversible. Where physical healing is apparently minimal, only internal healing makes meaning in life. Internal healing occurs when the afflicted person finds peace with a life that may not be the kind he anticipated. The body may still be broken, but the afflicted person is healed in his spiritual self, soaring with eagles. Chronic illness can be a stimulus to many kinds of internal growth that would have been not otherwise possible.

Healing comes rather easily when messages and meanings of illness are gently accepted.

Finding your spiritual self can help you separate emotionally from the disease itself and free you from the overwhelming feeling of 'I am my illness', which is always counterproductive. This is finding the wisdom at every moment by being fully present to one's spiritual self and the transcendent. The good way to take the sting out of life's painful experience is to seek the wisdom hidden in the challenge. For those who can do this, their lives will move forward; for those who cannot, bitter feelings and subsequent chronic illnesses usually happen. The Serenity Prayer is worth remembering as follows:

God grant me the serenity to accept the things I cannot change, courage to change the things I can, and wisdom to know the difference.

We need wisdom to become whole persons. From the holistic perspective, suffering comes from forgetting your wholeness. Any growth that frees us from the narrow consciousness of the individual ego is spiritual. Letting go of fear, worry, and stress – which is the matrix of our narrow ego consciousness – we connect ourselves to the healing power of the cosmic consciousness or that Higher Power of all spiritual traditions. Illnesses, crises, and sufferings are catalysts of spiritual growth. The crises and challenges we experience in our bodies are ultimately expressions of the spiritual self that want to evolve and grow to a higher realm.

When you find your spiritual self, you can separate yourself emotionally from the disease itself, which will impart to you a tremendous degree of empowerment. Discovering the spiritual self and experiencing it help us to disidentify ourselves with disease and the suffering attached to it. The healing process is enhanced when one is able to become impersonal about the presence of illness. This does not mean we are becoming incapable of emotions. Rather, it is aligning our emotions so that they may become supportive. It frees one from the overwhelming feeling of 'I am my illness' and similar preoccupations, which is negative and counterproductive.

Healing is transforming the areas of our lives that are not conducive to regain health. Every disease is a messenger, or a teacher, that helps you to understand some inner work to make life qualitatively rich and meaningful. Illnesses are often facilitators to effect qualitative changes in life. The messages, if well attended to, will direct one toward reevaluating one's identity, self, and its potential. It is the spiritual self that finds wisdom, meaning, and purpose in suffering and disease.

Holistic health attitudes or natural methods do not save individuals from illness. Exercise, yoga, meditations, natural foods, and natural lifestyles all help; still humans have to deal with the unpleasantness of disease. For, disease is a manifestation of evil in the body; and evil is a reality, at least in a world of relative experience. Management of its existence requires acknowledgement of its existence that sometimes requires suffering.[10]

Many lives have witnessed the fact that growth and transformation came to them due to their illness. Subsequently, they found meaning in their lives. To an outsider, it is an acute or chronic disease that added misery in life. Health problems challenge many to address the issues that they hitherto avoided. Spiritual growth and transformation are oftentimes the result of crisis, mostly in the form of disease.

Finding your spiritual self can help you separate emotionally from the disease itself and free you from the overwhelming feeling of 'I am my illness', which is always counterproductive.

Scientists may say nature is blind, meaningless, and purposeless. As we sometimes suppose, it is not indifferent. Nature, in its mysterious ways, always leads us to better health and meaning in life. Life is empowered when it finds meaning and purpose in life. It is an undeniable truth that suffering, illness, and experiencing the limitations of life led many to self-realization and healing. When people are confronted with disease, its pain and anguish nudges them to reconfigure themselves mentally and emotionally; and as a result of that, sometimes the body is healed. Illness can be a crucial and valuable opportunity to a more wholesome personality.

Healing involves radical changes in how you live and what you believe about yourself and life. Deep and lasting healing occurs when old habits and attitudes that led to the disease are cast off and replaced by healthy habits and attitudes. Pain and discomfort in the wake of illness are a correlation of activity of the nerves that are conveying information about the nature and extent of the injury to the brain that activates the mechanism for repair. Pain is intended to draw attention to that part of the body that needs attention. There is a symbolic meaning for our pain depending on the location where it appears.

Inner Freedom and Creativity

As human beings, we experience limitations in everyday life. To a great extent, we admit our limitations that come from external circumstances. But when one experiences limitations from within, the sense of limitation is overwhelming. The healing I envision comes when this sense of limitation is overcome. Healthy human beings are free to be active on three levels – physical, mental, and spiritual – to create and fulfill oneself and enrich others. A freedom of the body operates when none of the organs are limited and has no negative awareness of the bodily functions. The mental level is more critical for the human being than the physical realm, because it is on the mental realm that an individual thinks, criticizes, compares, calculates, visualizes, and communicates. Disturbances in this area take away from one's freedom and creativity, and thereby one's comfort and well-being.

A person can continue to be happy and, therefore, be creative for oneself and others with a crippled body, loss of limbs, loss of sight or hearing. In the history of mankind, many handicapped people lived fully without losing their freedom and creativity. Although the physical body is the medium through which the higher faculties are manifested in the material world, it can manifest powerfully even in the lesser bodily integrity. Physical debility, in itself, need not crush the creativity in the mental or spiritual plane until one gives in. The comparative degree of health one enjoys at a given time, if at all it can be distinguished, is by the creative freedom. Whether an individual with rheumatoid arthritis is in better health than another one suffering with depression is to be answered on the comparative degree of creative freedom. To the extent that an individual is limited in the exercise of creativity, to that degree he is ill. The state of mental and emotional health can be kept as long as one is altruistic, putting away selfishness and egotism.[11] Mental disintegration starts from possessive and acquisitive tendencies, which prompts oneself to pit one against another. By keeping a spiritual identity and awareness, one can disidentify oneself with things, people, and the world as well as the body and emotions. As a result, a serenity and calm will take hold on the mental plane, whereupon one will enjoy maximum freedom and creativity. In this manner of looking at health, the spiritual self is the primary 'gatekeeper' of our mental health and, thereby, physical health.

3

Symptoms, Diagnosis and Drugs

In my experience, someone rarely goes to a doctor to stay healthy. We are almost convinced that staying healthy is not the business of doctors and the medical profession. Your right to see a doctor is when you are sick, often seriously sick. In the old Chinese tradition, doctors were paid to keep patients healthy. So, if you were sick, the treatment was free. Keeping oneself healthy and sound is not the business of the doctor. They have not been trained to do so. They are taught to discern symptoms. When they identify a set of symptoms, they give a name to it and call it a diagnosis. If that is done, half of the problem is addressed. Once a diagnosis is made, it is much easier to deal with the case. Every disease is dealt with prescribing a drug or two, sometimes more than a half-dozen.

Symptom Language

Symptoms are the language of the body through which it sends warnings, messages and signals to repair the damaged mechanism. They are signals or warning signs telling you that something is wrong in your system. It is the end result in a series of occurrences going on in your system. Symptoms are the cry of nature to draw attention to your body when you have not been properly attending to it. People often fail to pay attention to their bodies until it hurts. Disease is a process that starts in the interior of the person. People sometimes go to doctors because they do not feel altogether well. They may not have a discernible symptom. They may feel weak, lack energy, and have little enthusiasm to engage in anything actively. In these instances, their health economy is suffering, but it has not become fully noticeable in terms of external symptoms. Nevertheless, the person is sick. If this initial state goes unheeded, it will then manifest itself from the level of the internal realm to the external realm.

Every investigation of a scientific character tells us that everything that exists does so because of something else existing prior to it. It is the individual's spiritual self that existed prior to the organs, tissues, and systems. No patient goes to the doctor and says 'my heart is sick' or 'my head is sick', but they will say 'I am sick.' Then, the doctor will review the sufferings the patient undergoes – the pain, the sleeplessness, the irritation, etc. From these numerous symptoms, the doctor arrives at an image of the sick person. However, it is not the image of the body part the doctor should draw upon, but primarily the sick individual himself. Symptoms are just indicators, telling us that the self is sick. Medical science recognizes nothing but the material principle and fails to notice the internal disorder. It focuses on the end process; that is, the symptoms, and arresting the symptoms. It is like killing the messenger because the news was bad. The messenger's message goes unnoticed or suppressed through the use of drugs and will usually manifest itself in a more distorted and gross form. Chronic diseases are mostly the failure to heed the message at the earliest time. Nature is there to help us: if we suppress nature, and simply use drugs so that it cannot speak to us, then we will have to pay a price for ignoring nature. Germs and microbes do not cause disease. It is the susceptibility of the host that makes the germs thrive. Every individual carries some level of virus, bacteria, and pathological element in the body. Generally, these factors do not cause any problems. They are the scavengers accompanying the disease. They are present whenever the interior of the person is sick or in disorganization. This internal principle is referred to in various philosophical traditions differently such as vital force, energetic principle, spiritual, etc.

It is rather easy to deal with what is visible and tangible. The invisible and transcendent parts of humans need more personal, committed attention and individual effort. So often, this part is easily overlooked. Leaving the primary cause and working on the secondary cause of disorders will not bring about healing in the patient. By arresting the symptom, the patient may be able to move through life and resume normal routines. Chest pain, difficulty in breathing, muscle and skeletal pain, dizziness, constipation, abdominal upset, insomnia, and fatigue are some of the complaints doctors often hear from patients. Yet, in three-quarters of these cases, doctors cannot find any existing disease. Doctors seek objective, measurable, and observable findings. However, in many instances, they do not find any. Yet, the person says he is sick, has a real problem and is suffering. The doctor insists on more tests, more experimental medication, and more appointments.

Symptoms have been the target of therapeutics. Modern medicine is incredibly skilled in suppressing symptoms without curing them.

Invasive procedures and drug therapies usually do not touch the core problem in the individual. The person may be cured but never feels he is quite the same as before. Throughout history, symptoms or a group of symptoms have been viewed as the real problem. Therefore, the fight has been against symptoms rather than against the disease.

Symptoms have been the target of therapeutics. A person who has a runny nose usually receives a decongestant; if constipated, a laxative; if there is pain, an analgesic. Conventional medicine never really considered the genesis and evolution of the disease but took only the final manifestation of the symptom. This did little to respect the symptom as an endeavor of the body to heal. Symptoms are the result of a lengthy process that already has entered into your system. People who are not in touch with their body sometimes never really know what has been going on inside of them until some alarm sounds in the form of an emergency.

Medicine generally suppresses symptoms without curing. We have impressive drugs that do the work. When symptoms are suppressed, no more alarms are sounded. Having no other outlet, the root cause of the stress now recedes to the interior plane of the individual. When you ignore the body's many smaller calls for attention, demanding little reassessment or reorganization of life from within and without, you build up a growing urgency that will lead to a major crisis of some sort. The growing epidemic of emotional and psychological problems of today's people mainly originates from suppressive medicines. Rudolph Ballentine in *Radical Healing* remarked: "Psychotherapy arose to replace the lost art of healing the body."[1]

The Nature of Healing

The body heals itself. It has an innate healing system. No outside agent or force can heal. Doctors and medicines can catalyze and bring about the healing response or remove obstructions to it. But, the body heals itself if we do not interfere with its healing process. Oftentimes, treatment and drugs interfere with the body's process of healing. Wound healing is a model for healing in general. In a healthy person, a wound that is clean and has bled freely will heal itself without the use of any medicine. The body takes its own time. A skin laceration takes little time to heal; a broken bone takes a longer amount of time. Again, some people heal faster than others. From very ancient times, people tended to rub wounds with strange substances, even using the excrement of animals. Oils, herbs, honey, and leaves all have been used in different geographical areas for the treatment of wounds.[2] Some of them might act as an antibiotic or antibacterial. Not much research has been done on any of these methods. As long as the chance of infection is reduced, any wound will heal naturally.

Good health is the intended state of the human being. Every aspect of our system is designed to fight forces that upset our health balance. Our healing system constantly monitors our body's cellular health. When its sensors detect a threat, warrior cells are sent to the area to meet the emergency. If you cut your finger, it starts bleeding, risking life through the loss of blood. But, it does not bleed limitlessly unless you aggravate it. The blood clots, or coagulates, and a scab is formed until healthy cells arrive, thereby preventing the exposure of the wound to infection. Break a bone in your leg and you will not be able to walk unassisted; you will need help for some period of time until the bone heals. But, as soon as your bone breaks, it starts to heal. Sometimes it needs your input or expert help depending on the gravity of the fracture.

The bone may need to be pushed back into the original position if it is displaced, and one must keep it in that position in order for it to be properly joined. What you have to do is to create the right conditions for the body to heal. Mentally and spiritually battered and abused people need more time to be healed. Even in those cases, recovery is the rule of nature. Not every individual who is abused lives a rotten and shattered life; they all recover over the years through therapy, support groups, or self-help programs. No one needs to be a victim forever. Healing is always a possibility. More serious health problems require a greater active role on the part of the individual concerned to obtain long-lasting health and recovery.

Healing involves three distinct components: reaction, regeneration, and adaptation. The inflammation that develops around the edges of a wound is an example of the reactive component of healing. Fever is another example. Fever helps the body fight infection. Most people think of inflammation and fever as an illness and aggressively treat them. This reactive phase may produce some discomfort, but it is important not to mistake these reactions for disease. They are primary symptoms of an underlying disease. Some of our tissues and cells have astounding regenerative capacity. Liver cells are amazing in their ability to make up for lost cells even if there is only half of the liver itself. But, in general, the more specialized a cell, the more its regenerative capacity is greatly reduced. Heart muscles and nerve cells in the brain are specialized cells and their losses are often irreparable. When reaction and regeneration cannot reverse the situation, the body resorts to adaptation and compensation. In the case of damaged heart muscles, to a certain extent, new pathways of circulation and electrical conduction may develop around the damaged area. Sometimes, the affected cells are sectioned off. Isolating the affected areas may prevent the disease from affecting other organs. Bodies can also wall off pockets of infection to form abscesses. This happens whenever the body's defenses cannot defeat the infection but are able to contain it. Greater adaptation is then seen at the behavioral levels. People who permanently lose an organ develop great adaptation. What is lost is compensated for in the remaining organs.

Health is not a static state. There is a dynamic state of equilibrium of different interacting forces and elements. So, it is not surprising that one feels variations in health. It is normal to lose health periodically in order to regain it. Whenever the equilibrium of the body breaks down, the body's innate healing system is on call to restore it. It operates continually, keeping most of us in good health in spite of illness and the forces of disorder that surround us constantly. Most illnesses are self-limiting because the healing system is able to handle them and restore the balance. So, generally speaking, healing is the rule of nature. Treatments, whatever the modalities, are intended to make right the atmosphere for the healing system and thereby facilitate the healing powers of the body. The best treatment is the least treatment – the least invasive, least drastic, least expensive – that activates spontaneous healing.[3]

Sometimes the healing system needs outside help to catalyze its work when certain stimuli are overpowering the healing system and its abilities. The symptoms request help in order to catalyze the body's system. Our immune system, which is not able to throw off an infection because of the sheer strength of the viruses or bacteria congregated in the system, needs help. Sometimes a toxic environment needs to be changed for the immune system to take hold. Sometimes the disturbing forces are so strong, they overwhelm the healing abilities of the body. Falling flat on the ground from a fifty-story building or being involved in a high-speed collision, death is the likely outcome. In such circumstances, the equilibrium of the body is overturned so that the healing mechanism finds itself to be totally inadequate.

According to George Vithoulkas, one of the world's leading practitioners and teachers of homeopathy, there are three factors that determine or alter the nature of a sickness: hereditary strength or weakness of the defense system; intensity of the morbific stimuli; and the degree of intensity by the suppressive treatment applied.[4] If the defense mechanism is weak, the center of gravity symptoms will tend to affect the deepest mental and emotional levels quite easily. If the defense mechanism is strong, the symptoms will continue on the least vital physical organs. The intensity of stimuli is received on the mental, emotional, and physical levels. If the shock to the system is very severe, even the strongest defense mechanism may not be able to maintain the equilibrium.

Sometimes, people with low vitality are unable to mount a sufficient healing response. A wound may not heal if there is a foreign matter in the wound in spite of all the best treatments. Likewise, any foreign element in the body's system, such as a powerful drug, renders healing impossible. It takes time for the body to throw off the toxins. At times, the body is not able to clean itself if the toxins are heavy and the cleansing system is heavily burdened. The digestive and circulatory systems must be sound in order to effect a good health response. We have seen earlier that psychological and spiritual stress can block healing. A great many factors are involved in the healing process. The body heals itself if you remove the obstacles and give it the right context.

Problems and Complexities of Diagnosis

Symptoms, diagnosis, and drugs are intimately-related concepts in medical science. Symptoms tell the doctor that the health of the patient is in a state of disorganization and needs to be remedied. Usually, the remedy is administered in the form of drugs or surgery. In order to determine the remedy, the doctor needs a diagnosis. In simple terms, it is the name given to the malady you suffer. Both doctor and patient want to know what the true nature of the disease is. Once you name something, it indicates that you have some control over it. Then, you are in a better position to handle that condition. For example, the military usually gives a name to their operation before they launch it. When a hurricane is predicted, a name is normally given to it before the government mobilizes the resources to defend the inhabitants against it. Where a health insurance system exists, the name of the disease treated is paramount in order to charge the insurance company.

Diagnosis is one of the main tasks of a physician. When a doctor makes a diagnosis, it is a feather in his hat and he assumes dignity and status. The diagnosis settles your curiosity regarding the nature of your disease. However, in more serious cases it may also unleash additional fears and anxiety. Oftentimes, a diagnosis is of no great help to patients. But, for the doctor, it is a relief. Now they can stop sweating. Now they know what to do. In the arsenal of *Materia Medica,* they know that they can find an array of drugs to target your problem. The sad thing is that the doctor who makes the diagnosis usually does not give much attention to the actual cause of your ill health. Once the diagnosis is made, actual causes go behind the scene. Suppose you are diagnosed for allergy or asthma; you will get some drugs based on the *Materia Medica*. However, the actual cause may be that you are allergic to dairy foods or living in a toxic environment.

Symptoms are the result of an ongoing malfunctioning process in the system, often interrelated. Heart disease is a multifactor problem arising from inflammation, insulin resistance, infections, depression, stress, lack of exercise, or nutritional deficiencies, etc. The doctor may give you a name for your heart troubles, such as *hypercholesterolemia*. However, it does not convey to you the real nature of your problem. When someone has diabetes, he may come down with various conditions such as high blood pressure, cataracts, arthritis, or kidney disease. Many diseases have a common thread, which oftentimes goes unnoticed.

The doctor cannot be much concerned about what causes the problem because he has more pressing things to do. He only needs to reduce your discomfort or pain and must remove you from the present endangerment. Finding out the real cause and building health is a much more committed, time-consuming, and disciplined task which neither the doctor nor the patient wants to do. According to a recent study in *The Journal of the American Medical Association*, the average interaction between doctor and patient lasts approximately twenty-three seconds without any interruption. In that amount of time, doctors can hardly pay full attention to all your symptoms. Before you are finished, they decide the treatment you need and, with pen and stationery, scribble out a recipe for you, which is best known as a prescription. Just because you are diagnosed with a disease, it does not tell you much about the problem, its true nature, or how to deal with it. It helps the doctor to come up with a prescription that might alleviate the immediate suffering of the disease and give some temporary relief. This necessarily does not have to happen because drugs, by their very nature, are not such simple substances that act as you may think.

Medical science operates from this general assumption: once there is a diagnosis, the patient needs some drug to cure the problem. So, you will see that doctors are quick to give you prescription drugs. The truth is that the conditions that affect most people these days are not necessarily diagnosable diseases because they are a combination of many causes, expressing themselves in various manners that elude diagnostic tools. Rudolph Ballentine, MD, a holistic clinician, regards the diagnosis as the major obstacle to enjoying the fruits of radical healing. "It is a wall. If you remain boggled by it, you will be severely limited in what you can do."[5] It is important to uncover the worldview that is the root of conventional diagnosis. The invention of the microscope led to the development of the germ theory of infection. With the discovery that germs are behind many diseases, such as smallpox, rabies, cholera, etc., medicine possessed an external scientifically-based cause of disease. People were no longer sick from within, but were being attacked by external agents over which one does not have much control. This led to a medical model that believes you become sick because something from the outside has attacked you, and it can be driven out or destroyed by some magic bullet called drugs.

Researchers have come up with claims that certain microbes are associated with cancer as well as arthritis.[6] Microbes may be present in many other diseases, too. The pertinent question is what appears first: microbes or the diseased tissue that invites them? Microbes are the by-products of a primary disorganization in the concerned system. Disorganization first occurs in the energetic and subatomic level. Any system is governed from the center to the circumference. For example, in the military, command centers control operations. Executive orders go from the command center to all other systems to be governed. The body and its operational systems are subjected to another higher command center. Materialistic medicine, by its bias, simply presupposes the ultimate cause of what happens is strictly on the physical level. It is part of a belief system that has both shaped and distorted the biological sciences. Unfortunately, the wisdom of the East and its philosophical and medical traditions were looked down upon by Western medicine.

There is an intense resistance in Western medicine to accept the power of the non-material. It holds almost a superstitious belief that only matter matters, and neither consciousness nor spirit are involved. Today, acupuncture is practiced throughout the world. Its medical efficacy is accepted nowadays almost everywhere. Science is in the pursuit of finding an explanation for its efficacy by ignoring the existence of the Chi energy in the body as is claimed by the acupuncture. With germs and microbes, the more subtle and invisible they become, the more powerful they can be in our system. This itself is an indicator that it is not the material reality that matters, but the subtle and invisible realms. The subtle energies of consciousness and the mind and its proper organization or disorganization affect the body system for good or bad that invite in the opportunist microbes and germs. Like acupuncture, homeopathy has been proven effective in many chronic cases and is based on the subtle energy patterns and its vibrations in our body.[7] Because medicine presupposes that the ultimate cause of what happens to us is on the physical level, cancer and arthritis are thought to begin in the tissues or joints.

The germ theory misses a key phenomenon that our 'biological terrain' is equally important in determining who becomes sick and how the illness progresses.[8] Every doctor holds a book as their Bible, namely *ICD.9.CM, The Diagnostic Classification for Medical Personnel*, with its 1,500 pages of diagnostic codes. Day-to-day medicine in hospitals, clinics, and labs around the world is designed to assess the symptoms and to make a diagnosis and treat them with drugs or surgery. The meaning of the symptom or its valuable information to the person concerned is never fully looked into or investigated. Because fear takes its grip at the onset of any symptom, we are only concerned about the enemy to be defeated with our medical technology and expertise.

Operating from fear, most people sabotage the healing from within. A vast majority reaches for suppressive medication for even a mild cold. Giving a little time for the body to heal is out of the question for many. They want a cure and need it now, instantly. The consumer culture has given us a mindset longing for instant pleasure without the checks and balances. It also reveals our increasing inability to delay instant gratification. Delaying gratification is a process of scheduling the pain and pleasure of life in such a way as to enhance the pleasure by meeting and experiencing the pain first and getting it over with.[9] Many are unwilling to put up with the temporary discomfort and inconveniences of the symptom. They rush to over-the-counter pills or to the doctor's office for a prescription.

Giving a little time for the body to heal is out of the question for many. They are looking for short-term relief more than actual healing.

The doctors run the risk of being unfairly accused of malpractice if they do not comply with the wishes of patients who ask for more and more analgesic pills to alleviate the discomfort. The patients demand instant cures and become irate if it is not provided to them. A certain level of pain is natural and should be endured during the period of recovery or healing. Sometimes, I am inclined to believe that people are looking for short-term relief more than actual healing that ultimately will make them well. Pills can in no way replace the needed attitudes and active role the individual has to play in the healing process.

Diagnosis is meaningful only when it gives you new information and understanding of what is going on in your body and connects the physical with the mental and energetic principles. We will have a more lengthy discussion on energetic principles later. In earlier periods, diagnosis was based on the patient's history and careful physical examination and asking the right questions in order to elicit the root causes. Lately, lab tests have supplanted all these methods. Doctors rely on instruments and procedures more than asking the right questions and making careful observations. With the emergence of high-tech diagnostic methods, diagnosis has become elaborate, invasive, and expensive. More and more, tests are now very routine such as a liver profile, a blood profile, etc. that doctors can order them without giving much thought to the underlying causes. There is a security aspect in so doing, for doctors are increasingly being sued for their sins of omission. Test results relieve them from responsibility to a certain extent. With the advent of extensive and expensive lab technologies, the doctor-patient relationship has dropped to its lowest point. You do not have to look to the patient but to the charts and test results. Everything gives the impression that doctors are highly scientific. However, the scientific dimension of the medicine does not capture the subtle things that are to be caught by observation and close bonding.

In diagnosis, the role of intuition cannot be overlooked. Experts in diagnosis always relied on their intuition, too. One of the pitfalls of relying too heavily on sophisticated diagnostic tools is often finding some abnormalities in one or another area of health. Health is not static but a dynamic interaction of different forces. In order to strike a balance in the system, the perfect health indicators may not always be present. A temporary shift in the balances can be expected in which the system will take care of itself. In the absence of a sound diagnosis, the patient with vague problems is likely to be tested again and again and be given experimental treatment to correct the disorder. Again, mechanical errors and handling errors are not uncommon. Invasive diagnostic methods make the patient more and more helpless and weak, creating a further need for intervention. Of course, some of the latest diagnostic procedures have life-saving dimensions and, as such, are indispensable. I am only pointing to the excessive reliance on these techniques in place of more simple methods that are safer, cheaper, and equally as helpful. Unfortunately, people also begin to think that the more expensive a treatment or more invasive it is, the more beneficial it should be. As technology takes its dominance, neither doctors nor patients make use of all their natural potential to maximize healing.

A New Worldview

Most people's worldview of reality is still that of the Newtonian era. In Newtonian physics, the mind and consciousness have no role. Quantum physics introduced us to a spectacular truth of ourselves and the world in which we live. We tend to and are taught to experience our body and world as solid matter. Quantum physics tells us that at the subatomic level, no matter exists but only an interconnection of energy waves. The energy waves' patterns and frequencies determine the final events. New physics contends that at the subatomic level, reality is determined and shaped by the observing mind. If there is no mind to observe or interfere in the subatomic field, the final event never comes to completion. It is the act of observation that brings a potential happening into a single result that can be called an actual event. If reality is tied to the observation of the mind that observes and interferes, then it can impact the phenomenon it observes. That means by your intentionality and by your process of observation, you can change the final reality. A process – your malady – that is set in motion within your body can be affected by the way you want to observe it. The symptom one observes in the body is part of a dysfunctional process that is progressing to a finality. Symptoms are indications of a process in the body which are yet to be determined. It has not yet become a final reality.

When scientists observe the universe from a quantum perspective, they find in every fabric of space and time an all-pervading force. They have discovered that this force is spread throughout the universe in an infinite wave – the quantum wave. The universal glue or factor that holds it all together can be called the universal consciousness or Universal Self.[10] Just as larger universal consciousness holds and shapes the quantum waves according to its intelligence and plans, at the human level, it is the human consciousness that shapes and forms the immediate reality subjected to the intelligence of the universal consciousness. So, what we choose to think, observe, and learn is important whether it be in matters of health or disease. Our health and illnesses are flexible and susceptible to being shaped by our consciousness.

Physicist Helmut Schmidt's studies over many years and the experiments he conducted indicate the likelihood that humans can mentally influence the behavior or output of random event generators.[11] Schmidt's contention is that past subatomic events are malleable, capable of being influenced mentally, even though they have already occurred as long as they have not been consciously observed. Schmidt's observations have wider implications to the health field. Many diseases begin with disturbances at the subatomic level. While disease appears to be in the whole organs such as the lungs, heart, or kidneys, their most fundamental sight of origin is in the subatomic field. This gives us the possibility to change the subatomic field that is already in process. The process can be reversed or changed by the mind that enters into the field. If the behavior of the subatomic particle is associated with disease causation, we may be able to redirect its behavior in order to bring about health. Quantum physics holds the view that observing and looking convert possibilities and potentialities into actual events and fixes them irrevocably.[12]

Taking to heart the maxim "Prevention is better than the cure," a good number of people subject themselves to annual medical exams. Periodic checkups make sense because they may uncover problems before they become manifest. A cancerous lump discovered at an earlier stage can be removed without invoking a major complication. Likewise, if diabetes is discovered at the early stage, the heart, kidneys, and blood vessels can be protected from further harm for many years. However, even with all the precautionary checkups, there is little evidence that health problems have significantly decreased in the past decade. Taking medical tests, accepting the diagnosis, and beginning a treatment are very critical factors. By taking these actions, you are defining your disease once and for all. Sometimes you may accept a verdict that you can change or you may keep it afloat indefinitely.

When the doctor defines a disease with a diagnosis, its nature is not finally decided until you accept, observe, and consciously take it to heart.

As long as things remain unobserved and unexplored or not studied closely, the fate of the disease is not firmly fixed. I have seen the health situation of many people deteriorate soon after the diagnosis. And, one then wonders how did they live all these years with the disease in their body? The dictum – if you have once been to the doctor, you are going to be doing it for the rest of your life – assumes greater implications when looking at it from this angle. What I am opposed to is not paying attention to the body and defining the messages the body sends. We have certain control over the health and healing process within the parameters of our nature and consciousness. Sometimes, the delay of a diagnosis and use of drugs can also delay a downhill course of the illness. My own experience has helped me to come to this conclusion.

I had been following a healthy lifestyle ever since I took interest in holistic medicine. I believed I had the perfect diet. When I turned 45, my friends advised me to have a medical checkup knowing my family history of heart disease. I remarked that I did not need a medical checkup since I followed a natural lifestyle. I refused to consider the possibility that I could have a problem with cholesterol, high blood pressure, or insulin resistance in the near future. After hearing of one more episode of heart failure and death within my family, my relatives pressured me by saying that my holistic practices alone could not save life, and that I should immediately go for a checkup. I did go this time. In the checkup, I found to my shock that I had a high cholesterol count of 270. The doctor advised me to watch my diet. I stated that I didn't know how much I could do by means of diet; still I indicated that I would try. Because I did not want to take any pills, I watched my diet very carefully. I wanted to see after three months time what amount of reduction I could make in the cholesterol count. I went to the lab for the test. When the results came back, I was disappointed. My cholesterol count reached 310! I could have never imagined that result. I did not believe it. I looked for another lab, but it showed the same result, more or less. I began taking Lipitor to lower my count, which reduced it by twenty-five percent during a six-month period, and then I stopped taking the drug. I did not go in for a test for three years. I took my focus off from the issue and moved on, not being concerned about it. My recent blood test shows my total cholesterol count to be 270, which is where I began, and I have come to the conclusion that it is natural to me. I believe the medical tests and diagnosis led me to make a close study and observation of the process in the subatomic level that defined the process hitherto not defined. The process in my system began at an earlier date and assumed a finality with the tests and diagnosis. If nothing had been done, and things were left as is, it would have delayed the progress to a finality. Diagnosis is a much-acclaimed tool in the medical field. It is helpful for the doctors, as we have noted earlier, to come up with a treatment plan. When physicians are unable to make a speedy diagnosis, they may feel they are inadequate. The patient often feels that he has fallen into a pit where even the doctor cannot come to his aid. Unfortunately, hardly anyone passes through life without undergoing at least a dozen or so medical tests.

Even after a diagnosis, some people refuse to accept the verdict of having a serious problem. In their denial, they do not pay close attention to the newly found reality. By not affirming it and refusing to admit it, one can stop giving control over to the disease. You may be able to push on and make progress more than medical science says. There have been many instances where people have been restored to health. There is a period of time that elapses before a disease is irrevocably decided. It is the time from symptom appearance, to diagnosis, to the beginning of treatment. This defining time is accelerated by medical procedures. Other than in cases of acute medical care and emergencies, less medical intervention is probably good. You will become more convinced about this as you familiarize yourself with the world of drugs. People who outlive medical statistics and predictions are often those who refuse to buy into the standard diagnostic labels attached to them by the medical world.

Drugs or Remedies

Although the words *medicine* and *drugs* are being used interchangeably, each has its own nuance. In the whole medical field, we have only a few substances that can be called ***medicine.*** It is a particular substance for a particular disease: a one-to-one application that can effectively eradicate the problem without side effects or jeopardizing other functions and the vitality of the patient; such medicines are rare in conventional medicine. So, it is better that we say most substances are medicinal rather than a medicine. The word *remedy* is often used to refer to more natural agents, such as herbs and homeopathics. Drugs are chemical compounds designed to alter metabolic reactions. They give some symptom relief as they interfere with the targeted biochemical process in the body. They oftentimes upset the whole balance of the body. The drug acts harshly on the system as a foreign element that the body never accepts. The body is being pushed around by the chemical power of the drug. The drug pushes its way into the system disregarding the body's own healing efforts. It does not cooperate with the healing system the body possesses; rather, it interferes with it and pushes its own agenda on a targeted field. The patient feels this struggle in the whole system whenever he takes a gross drug. People usually can feel in their very being the struggle between an impulse within and the chemical drug. Orthodox medicine prefers substances that cause immediate, dramatic changes, even at the expense of much greater side effects. Drugs, by their arbitrary function, cover up or thwart the expression of the disease. Therefore, they are not healing. It is a kind of disease management for temporary relief. Remedies, on the other hand, are substances chosen to address the underlying problem. They correct the imbalances in the energy flow and its patterns. They act more on the subtle and molecular level. Correct remedies will bring out the disorder or symptoms fully so that you can know its exact nature and can address it squarely by knowing its nature. A remedy shall not suppress or cover up symptoms.

Finding the right informational package is the task of a natural healer. Nature is there to help us always in many different ways. The Doctrine of Signatures has been a valuable tool and pointer to the remedies in the past centuries. Physicians and philosophers attempted to determine the therapeutic effect of drugs through the Doctrine of Signatures. By the Doctrine of Signatures, the intrinsic qualities of plants were studied – the color, appearance, shape, and other botanical features – including growth patterns. Their habitats were natural pointers to the likely curative value of the plant extracts. Nature has provided the means for mankind to cure most of its ills, and it is for man to seek and find it out without bias and preconceived notions. Homeopaths extended the Doctrine not only to the plant kingdom but also to the animal and mineral kingdoms. I would like to point out two examples to illustrate this point.

Pulsatilla Nigricans is a plant grown in clusters in the open space. This is a very mild gentle plant yielding to the winds. It suffers easily from the heat and cold. The little plant is shy and unobtrusive, popping up from year-to-year in varied locations in a field or garden. These specifications tell us the type of person and the illness it can cure. Rarely, one can find it growing as a single plant. That tells us of its gregarious nature. The Pulsatilla has a supple stem that bends with the wind. It survives because it is flexible and yielding. In fact, its other name is Wind Flower. In the same manner, Pulsatilla-type individuals are usually chilly and dislike the cold as well as sitting in the sun. The Doctrine of Signatures indicates that these people will be mild and yielding, readily give way to avoid any unpleasantness. The plant blooms in April and May, not in the heat of summer. Our physical, mental, and spiritual nature is also reflected in the natural world of plants, minerals, and animals.

In another example, the very physical nature of phosphorous tells us that such a person will be less likely to be a materialist. Phosphorous, when exposed to air, vaporizes and disappears leaving no trace. The Doctrine of Signatures indicates that phosphorous-type individuals live on a higher intellectual plane; are imaginative, artistic and clairvoyant. The skin complexion of a phosphorous patient is variously described as sickly or waxy. They easily flush and have an unquenchable thirst, which is another feature of this type of person. I believe nature is always there to help us in our growth and well-being, if we honor the lessons that nature gives us. There is no reason to disregard this Doctrine that has been clinically observed over the centuries. If we accept the tips of nature, we will grow with nature towards a greater well-being. Homeopathy relies greatly on this ancient wisdom to find the constitutional medicine for each individual.

Quantum physics and Eastern philosophies tell us that everything in life is connected. We are not isolated units acting independently; everything interacts with everything else in varying degrees. We are all part of a quantum field. We are all a representation of one and the same energy appearing in different forms. We are each an integral part of the universe's web of energy-related events. At the subatomic level, there are no distinctions between our being and every other form of being in the universe. Therefore, you are reflected in nature and nature is reflected in you. We say man is a microcosm of nature. This interpenetration of nature helps us to find curative medicines.

The plants, minerals, or other substances that contain elements of your nature have a power to reprogram your energetic system. When you receive the right information nature has designed for you, you experience a sudden shift as if everything in the body reorganizes itself. When you take an aspirin, your headache goes away; it is because the acetylsalicylic acid is blocking certain pain-causing substances and messengers. It is not the result of a repatterning of your mental, emotional or energetic function that does away with the chain of events that is responsible for the experience of pain.

Drugs – Use and Abuse

The field of medicine is complex and is changing rapidly. Every day new clinical studies come out with far-reaching consequences in the administration and application of therapeutics. It is hard to keep up with all the new information. And, it is often confusing for professionals not to inform the laymen of these findings. Caffeine, chocolates, and eggs, which previously have been considered detrimental to health, are now considered as having some beneficial effects; so avoiding them altogether is not good for you either. Research methodologies and motivations sometimes are not fully justified. There are many inferior researches out there. So, sometimes a little personal observation, experience, and common sense make more sense than research findings.

If you must make a visit to the doctor, you naturally expect to receive some prescriptions; if you do not receive one, you will be disappointed. Many patients look down upon a doctor who does not prescribe some medication. They might even think of switching to another doctor. The dispensing of drugs has been woven into the very fabric of modern medicine. Taken a step further, the word *medicine* has become a synonym for the pharmaceutical product.

It is shocking to note that the word *drug* comes from a Greek word referring to poison. All drugs are poison in high enough doses. That is why drugs are administered with great care, as prescribed by the doctor and dispensed by a licensed pharmacist. Toxicity from a drug is a great problem. When one is sick, our systems are overburdened, weak, and not functioning properly. The advantages of a little symptom relief are often discredited by the long-term toxicity that remains in the body and the subsequent problems it creates. Since immediate relief for the patient is the main objective for all concerned, little time and effort is spent on the long-term effects or side effects of the drug. An adverse drug reaction accounts for the vast majority of iatrogenic illness.[13] It can be anything mild, ranging from nausea, headache, drowsiness, hives or serious damage to any organ or system.

Most of the drugs administered are detrimental to health. According to a 1998 study in *The Journal of the American Medical Association*, adverse reaction to prescription drugs ranks as the sixth leading cause of death in United States. Because our bodies have tremendous adaptability, most of us survive despite ingesting these foreign materials into our body. In excess, it upsets the balance of the healing system upon which you will find yourself taking more and more medicine, each one for different reasons. When drugs take control, the healing system ends up in disarray, and the body becomes helpless in building good health. Drugs induced will be giving some symptom relief for a short time, whereas your health is never returned or restored to its former state. The average patient in a hospital is placed on a half-dozen drugs simultaneously. Little research has been done on the interactions of the drugs administered as one unit. Doctor's information on the majority of cases about the toxicity and side effects are drawn from pharmaceutical companies who obviously want to promote their products. Everybody knows of the unhealthy connection between the pharmaceutical industry and the doctors and hospitals. The techniques of persuasion and gift giving among these professions are outrageous.

In countries where advanced medicine and its administration save people and promote health, it would be staggering to hear about the astronomic number of errors and blunders that complicate life or kill people. The 1994 December issue of *The Journal of the American Medical Association* acknowledges 180,000 deaths occur every year at hospitals by means of errors. In spite of all these odds, medical science still enjoys credibility and power because it can solve problems in acute cases. When you are bleeding in an accident with broken bones and writhing in pain, you badly need medical science and its skills. Whoever comes to us in acute need is embraced as the savior. So, medical science is looked upon as a savior who can restore health. Since it has not taken into account the whole human person when dealing with everyday health problems and chronic illnesses, medical science has woefully failed.

New research and findings in the field of health almost everyday contradict what has been held earlier. The search for links between diet, lifestyle and environmental factors has not taken us anywhere we feel safe. It only has added further confusions to health-conscious people. At one time, fat was the main villain behind most health problems and obesity; now it is carbohydrates. Coffee and alcohol were always bad for you; however, now experts say when taken in moderation they are good. Hormone replacement therapy (HRT) was considered very normal and benevolent at one time; now women are warned against its dangerous side effects. Studies now tell us mammography does not add much to protect women from breast cancer. Doctors prescribe aspirin to most heart patients to ward off further stroke or heart attack. It has been taken faithfully by many patients. A new study appeared recently that suggests aspirin does little for many heart patients. Most patients are either non-responsive or resistant to aspirin. That means aspirin does not have the desired effect on the blood for many of the pill takers. Doctors hardly check for resistance or non-responsiveness. It is administered routinely.

Diabetic patients are treated with higher and higher doses of insulin on the premise that there is an insulin deficiency. In a good number of cases, it is not the lack of insulin but the body's inability to respond to the insulin. Adding more insulin may only jack up the blood pressure and create subsequent problems. In the short term, raising insulin will lower blood sugar. However, over time these drugs stop working because the body gets dependent on it and becomes resistant to it. The higher level of insulin administered to lower the blood sugar level has been shown to increase heart disease, the main cause of death in diabetic patients. When the problem is too much insulin and the increased resistance to it, adding more insulin shots is shooting at the wrong target. The key to restore the body's sensitivity to insulin is to avoid drugs, change diet, control weight, and exercise regularly. Generally speaking, patients as well as doctors look for quick fixes and quick results. Health and healing is the by-product of lifestyle, attitudes, values, outlook, etc. It is not produced or lost in a moment other than when we meet with a catastrophic accident or something of that sort.

Drugs are expert in disrupting and disorganizing, whereas nature's remedies are gentle as they are meant to reorganize and reprogram our whole body's functioning. Drugs lack the subtle and needed information to correct the imbalances. They can help to buy time. In a crisis situation, a person may have to rely on drugs to tide one over the crisis. It seems evident to common sense that as nature supplies all the food we need to nourish a healthy life, it should also supply all the remedies for diseases.[14] Every animal apparently knows its own remedy, and from man's observation of animals and what they do when they are sick, there is a telling example of the value of nature to cure us from afflictions. Science has slowly realized that all the chemical elements we need, of which our bodies are composed, are contained in the roots, barks, leaves, flowers and the fruit of herbs. Each family of plants has its own peculiar habit of taking from the soil special groups of chemical elements. The family called legumes – peas, beans, and cloves – gives calcium, potassium, phosphorous, etc. in a non-poisonous form. Lime plants present us with material to build bone, ligaments, and teeth, etc. There are iron plants that supply food for blood, and phosphorous plants that supply food for the brain and nervous system. It is unlikely that our body's living cells can benefit substantially from the inorganic, synthetic, and artificial substances.

The year 1803 witnessed a critical development of synthetic drugs as we know them today. At that time, a German pharmacist, Friedrich Wilhelm Sertürner, isolated morphine from opium. It led to the extraction of the active substances from plants and herbs. The extraction of the active principle from the crude plant made its administration very easy. Now, you could measure the quantities and qualities of the substance unlike in the crude plant form. A good number of drugs are made out of plants. One might then think that the extracted drugs have all the benefits of the natural plant's power to heal. However, it is a mistaken notion. Drug plants are complex mixtures of chemicals, all of which contribute to the effect as a whole. The more active principle need not in itself have all curative effects. Drug plants differ from the pure compounds that are derived from them. Isolated and refined drugs are much more toxic than their botanical counterparts. They tend to produce effects of a more rapid onset, greater intensity, and shorter duration. Sometimes they fail to produce the desirable actions of the plant, and they are likely to lack the natural safeguards when used as a part rather than as a whole.[15] The excessive use of drugs in allopathic medicine is its worst sin.

Antibiotics, although necessary and lifesaving at times, are frequently overprescribed. This has led to extreme antibiotic resistance in many people. Every course of action taken by the use of antibiotics makes the body inhabited by a more resistant organism. Frequent use of antibiotics kills many beneficial bacteria that balance the various internal systems. Sometimes antibiotics are given to prevent problems before any infection arises. It is a kind of overuse of the medicine because the toxicity interferes with the healing process. It is not preventive medicine when it is overused.

People who travel from country to country sometimes complain about having stomach problems. When you travel, your body takes in different kinds of food and water from totally different environments. Germs and bacteria differ from place to place, and they are present in every food and drink. Far from causing trouble, they live in harmony with the host and in balance with the intestinal cells, enabling them to digest food. Our intestines do contain bacteria, which helps in digestion and produces elements needed for maintaining our system and immunity. These bacteria differ from place to place. Food from a new environment with different kinds of organisms disturbs the existing balance. It will take time for the body to adjust to the new organisms. When we travel, our intestines are faced with new bacteria. Our intestines have to strike a new balance with these new bacteria in order to function harmoniously in the new milieu. This balancing is a slow process. If you take rest and do not stress your system further by heavy food, it will take care of itself. If you take an antibiotic, it may make things worse.

> ***Drugs are experts in disrupting and disorganizing the body's healing system. None of the drugs solve the basic problem, but save you from the immediate crisis.***

When the cure is within our reach, rushing for antibiotics or drugs is doing violence to one's body. Antibiotic treatments often aggravate digestive problems by changing the delicate balance of bacteria in the stomach. The beneficial bacteria in our intestines, such as lactobacillus and bifidabacteria, perform chemical transformation such as synthesizing vitamins and nutrients. They manufacture vitamin K, some B-vitamins, and produce certain molecules that have anti-cancer properties. These bacteria have an excellent symbiotic relationship with us by which both parties thrive. The stress we place on our intestines because of the use of alcohol, sugar, and antibiotics very often disturbs the normal ecological balance of the gastrointestinal system causing certain bacteria to grow unchecked.

Antibiotics are needed to fight in critical cases. It is important to remember that drugs do not solve the basic problem. The patient still needs to find out what has created the problem and must identify and address those issues for true healing to occur. Antibiotics are likely to make the individual susceptible down the road to further problems. Despite its drawbacks, antibiotics are life saving when serious infection occurs in vital organs. Until recently, women's symptoms related to menopause were treated as a disease. The symptoms such as hot flashes, night sweats, and sleep disturbance were diagnosed as being caused by a lack of estrogen. So, the common treatment given was a hormone replacement therapy (HRT) in the form of estrogen. Millions of women in the Western world were administered an estrogen drug called Premarin. It took three decades to come to the realization that the estrogen level does not actually decline until a woman has stopped menstruating altogether, and even then most women produce some amounts of estrogen. Without any discernment, however, almost every woman with menopausal symptoms was administered an estrogen replacement drug. This resulted in an increase in the number of breast and uterine cancer cases, blood clots, gallstones, high blood pressure, fibroids, migraines, weight gain, and even strokes and heart attacks. Who spread the myth that estrogen replacement is indispensable for the health of women? The powerful pharmaceutical industry. It is common knowledge that large insurance and pharmaceutical companies and medical associations often influence trends in the medical field.

The toxicity of drugs is often rated by a number called the therapeutic ratio: a ratio of the minimum dose producing toxic effects to the minimum dose producing the desired effects. For many drugs in current use, that number is between 10 and 120. This number is equivalent to ten times the dose of aspirin used to relieve a headache – sufficient enough to cause symptoms of salicylate poisoning. The pharmacological industry and doctors prefer increased potency, power, and rapid action for the drugs they administer. There is a widespread ignorance among physicians about the effects and interactions of the drugs they use. Voltaire remarked long ago, "Physicians pour drugs of which they know little, to cure diseases of which they know less, into humans of which they know nothing."

Louis Pasteur's theory and practice led everyone to believe that microbes are the cause of illness. As the result of that theory, the science of bacteriology made rapid advancement. Antibiotics became the main armor against infectious diseases. Penicillin and other antibiotics could check the contagious diseases and some major killers of the times such as tuberculosis, syphilis, and pneumonia. The power of antibiotics in the case of some diseases made everyone think that there is an external cure for every disease. The materialistic philosophy of allopathy ignored all other causative agents of illness and focused on microbes. Thus, the overuse of antibiotics flourished in the field of medicine. People are no longer sick from within but were being attacked by external factors. The germ theory missed a key factor called the "biological terrain"

– that is our total being – in determining who became sick and how the illness progressed. Slowly, medicine now has come to acknowledge that the microbe and constitution susceptibility of the individual are necessary to incite the disease process. The obsession with microbes led researchers far from the real causative factors of illness. The vast majority of drugs prescribed for illnesses such as arthritis, asthma, heart disease, epilepsy, anxiety, and depression are not designed to be curative even in their original concept.[16] They do not strike at the root of the illness but merely offer some palliation with total disregard for side effects. Technological advancement in the medical field has fascinated people and gives the impression that everything is scientific, modern, and up-to-date.

Suppressive medications for minor colds, coughs and rashes have become commonplace. We saw that symptoms are messengers that carry important information. Each time suppressive medications are ingested, symptoms go deeper into the system from the peripheral. Since it is then not allowed to operate on the periphery without affecting vital organs and systems, it assumes a more subtle character and goes inside to the interior economy of the individual, affecting the whole person. More and more drugs mean a weaker and weaker healing system and its defenses. Immunity from symptoms is not a sign of improved health but degeneration in the ability of the person to send any new messages out. This is what we call chronic disease. The whole person's life and being is now affected. The alarming rate of chronic diseases could be the result of suppressive therapies.[17]

So many wonder drugs have been marketed over the past decades. Most of them are lifestyle drugs – treatments that target issues of comforts, convenience, and appearance. Consumers can be confused by the ever-widening array of health products competing for their attention and money. Commercials are driving consumers to buy more expensive drugs or unnecessary drugs than they actually require. Sadly, consumers do not get sufficient information to make a best judgment regarding whether the marketed and advertised products are delivering any real value. Sometimes people think an expensive drug is more effective than a low-cost drug. After making a diagnosis, the next natural step for a physician is usually to prescribe a medication, hardly asking questions about diet, exercise and lifestyle. What is most inexcusable is prescribing a medication for a symptom that is most likely caused by another medication already prescribed. There is no incentive for doctors to promote well-being. They are trained to diagnose and prescribe according to the symptoms present.

Excessive Surgeries

We cannot think of a life without allopathic medicine and its surgical skill. Medicine has become a new religion. Modern medicine is effective in dealing with many serious problems. In the wake of an accident, you need a modern hospital and high-tech labs. There are acute surgical emergencies such as hemorrhages in the brain, intestinal blockages, urinary obstructions, etc. With all its merits, modern medicine has its disadvantages, too, many of which could be avoided by looking for other resources. Until recently, allopathy was the only form of medicine taken seriously.

People were enamored by the power of drugs and the surgery that can turn lives around. The surgical power of medicine goes back to the earliest attempts to deal with wounds. The art of surgery grew in leaps and bounds because of war and the need of care for the wounded, debilitated and dying. Surgery has rescued many millions from immediate death. Accident victims have been greatly helped by surgeries. Many mothers and babies have been saved from certain death of birth problems. Vital organs permanently damaged such as the heart, kidney, or liver are now replaced by surgery. Many are now able to enjoy health and life on account of such surgeries. Humanity has drawn numerous benefits from surgical medicine.

Cosmetic surgery has also helped many people whose injury or natural defects prevented them from becoming effective people in society. I have marveled at the skills of surgeons who can make life and death differences in the lives of people. As like in any good thing, unfortunately, we have also witnessed a lot of abuse in this area. Instead of making surgery a last resort when all other things fail, many surgeons go ahead with surgery as their first option. Scarcely any patient will defy the recommendation of their surgeon. Unnecessary surgery is commonplace today, such as removing one's appendix, tonsils, uterus, or breast. Not all organs and their precise functioning are clear to modern medicine. Earlier, the pineal gland, located in the center of the brain, was considered practically useless and surgeons dared to remove it. It took time to realize that it is the master gland of the endocrine system, regulating biorhythms and hormonal cycles. Surgeons themselves will agree that twenty-five percent of all surgery is unnecessary. This was observable, in particular, at the time of a doctors' strike, when practically all routine surgery patients were put on hold, while only emergency surgery went on unchanged. Analysts found less adverse medical incidents and death during such periods. It is always desirable to seek a second opinion when drastic measures are recommended by any doctor. Invasive surgeries on a healthy body, that can survive the crisis in its own way with little input from the patient, will do much harm to the health system. Surgeons, by the very nature of their profession, are inclined to propose surgery most times.

Surgeons enjoy mythical powers. They can put you into a sleep-death state and bring you back again to life. They enjoy the power to stop the heart and re-start it again. People naturally have faith in the astounding magical power of surgeons and surgery. The successful and more serious surgeries always boost the image of surgeons in the medical community as well as among the public. More people will be seeking the surgeon who performed it. After all, more surgery means more prestige and more money.

Many people begin to look upon surgery as a quick panacea for their many ills. The increase in the alarming rate of surgery speaks for itself that practitioners as well as patients are simply ignorant of the basic principles of health. The impression medicine created that there is a ready-made solution for health problems, either in the form of drugs or surgery, has led people to shirk the responsibility of maintaining good health and preventing serious disease. Studies reveal that coronary bypass surgery for angina and coronary artery disease have only a minimal advantage.[18] It may be able to buy some additional time, but the risk of further arterial disease, and possibly death from a heart attack, may not change. Most surgeons and physicians are well-meaning people, but blind faith in themselves, technology, drugs and surgery to the exclusion of other considerations can lead to destructive results. Any medical procedure can bring change and better health, depending on many other factors such as the placebo effect and belief system of the patient.

4

Health and Belief System

It is not an exaggeration to say that one's belief system has the power to unlock or lock healing energies. This is an area that presents many possibilities. In the past decades, studies and research are stunning. It challenges us to re-evaluate and assess some of our cherished notions and conceptualizations in the medical field. We create reality by our values, beliefs and worldview. My world and its experience are shaped by what I believe to be true. Faith and beliefs will eventually be translated to physical realities. It is my interior world of ideas, values, and faith that decide the quality of my life.

The Power of Beliefs

Sometimes, strong affirmative beliefs are all one needs to be healed. At other times, creating a conducive physical environment by means of medicine or surgery is essential along with other beliefs. Since it is difficult to measure how much one's belief system helps and what percentage medicine helps, it is desirable to promote the belief system. Promoting positive beliefs and confidence in oneself (the power of one's body to heal), a doctor and medicine can affect healing, whereas one element taken by itself may fail. Humans have always entertained beliefs in oneself, nature, God, and in other people who can take care of them. At times, belief is shaken by certain accidents or disasters, but sooner or later, the individual regains it again. The sooner one regains it, the better that one can build up one's health. Lack of faith in oneself, in a Transcendent Being, and in others means losing the vitality of life. A belief system shaken means life's energy ebbs. In the final analysis, depression is a loss of faith in oneself, nature, and the Transcendent. Life's energy bounces back when faith is regained.

We are wired to believe. Beliefs can be rational and scientific. Most times, it need not be rational and scientific. The power of your belief is not dependent upon how much objective truth is in your thoughts and beliefs. A 1998 study conducted at Brown University by Dr. John F. Reilly and his colleagues found that patients with chronic pain often find themselves experiencing chemical dependence, emotional distress, and marital and family disruption. They express a disability pervading in all aspects of their lives. It is not the pain itself that impairs their life and its mobility, but the belief that pain has twisted and distorted their lives. The belief begins to work in their system as a self-fulfilling prophecy.

> ***The intensity of the belief matters when it comes to healing and health. Whether your faith is scientific or irrational, once you believe, it can trigger certain biochemical realities within your body.***

Since a belief was not measurable and tested, science tended to overlook its positive and negative impact. You can choose to have beliefs and thoughts that are beneficial for health and well-being. Our basic beliefs are the springboard of our continuous thoughts and images. Beliefs color our interpretation of the world; they affect our behavior. We create a world based upon our beliefs.

Hundreds of different therapies are being practiced throughout the world to effect cure. Some of them are inconsistent with the principles of any healing. In spite of these glaring defects, certain therapeutics could effect cure. It is obvious that it is not the therapeutic principles involved in the medicine system that heals, but something else. Those who choose certain types of therapeutics prefer them because of their strong belief in them. This belief in a therapeutic system is important in healing. Practitioners who can create a belief in their system, though objectively it may be unsound, can cure patients. As long as the therapy is professed to be the latest and the greatest, a vast majority of patients will experience excellent results. As soon as the patient's faith in the therapy is gone, the results also fade. What we believe about our doctors and medical treatment will markedly affect our illness and recoveries. A number of studies have revealed that a patient's faith in the therapeutics and a higher expectation in the doctor's skill and expertise, as well as the doctor's own confidence and enthusiasm, can alleviate a variety of medical conditions including angina, asthma, herpes, cold sores, and duodenal ulcers.[1] Some practitioners are effective therapists because of the way they relate with patients. The relationship itself becomes therapeutic. A practitioner's faith in his therapeutics excites the patient's belief. The patient then easily takes on the doctor's confidence. So, the patient's faith, the practitioner's faith, and the relationship that exists between the patient and the therapist are the three principles involved in any healing besides the efficacy of any medicinal intervention.

Doctor-Patient Relationship

Dr. Herbert Benson's studies found that the patients who received friendlier, supportive visits recovered faster and were discharged earlier from the hospital an average of 2.7 days than patients in the control test group.[2] Patients treated in a warm and sympathetic manner experienced less pain, asking for half as much pain-alleviating medicine compared to those in a control test group. In 1987, a study published in the *British Medical Journal* examined the effects of the doctors' conveyance of positive or negative information to two hundred patients with symptoms not attributable to any particular physical ailment. In the positive consultations, the doctors gave patients an assured diagnosis, confidently remarked that the ailment would not need any prescription, and that they would feel improvement within a few days. To other patients, doctors gave prescriptions with confidence and very encouraging words. In fact, the prescriptions were really vitamins. In the negative sessions, the physician said that he was not sure of the nature of this ailment. However, he would give the patient a prescription that may help. Again, in fact, it also was a vitamin. The patients were told they could return to the clinic for more detailed observation if they did not get better. In the end, sixty-four percent of the patients who heard good news got better within two weeks of their consultation compared to only thirty-nine percent of those who received negative feedback. The weight of the doctor's words was proven all the more consequential because statistically there was little difference between those who received prescriptions and those who did not. No matter how successful the surgery, you will recover more speedily if your surgeon is confident, supportive, and upbeat. Confidence and faith can be instilled by caregivers and doctors by forging a trusting relationship if it is lacking in the patient. A physician's reassurances can make the physiological difference. Our attitudes and belief systems affect people close to us. A doctor's beliefs, personality, and behavior patterns affect the way in which the patients are treated and healed.

All kinds of healers enjoy an aura associated with healing powers. They are usually held in high esteem as if they possess some magical power. They keep up this aura by mystifying the nature of the disease. The faith of the patient in his healer has worked most of the time. However, the simple reassurance of healers does not work these days because people are inclined to look for facts and figures, as well as the credentials and expertise of the doctor. The doctor-patient relationship has suffered a great deal because of sophisticated technologies. Patients are interacting more with machines than with personnel in the hospital milieu.

Why Not More Placebos?

By definition, a placebo is an inert substance – mostly a sugar pill – designed to look like a real drug and given to satisfy the desire of the patient for medicine when no indication exists for a genuine prescription. Generally speaking, patients who go to the doctor expect some kind of medication for their cure. For, the common belief is that medicine means a cure. Consequently, no medication means no cure. Patients believe that medicine, at the very least, is good to speed up the cure. Everyone goes to hospitals and clinics with this or similar beliefs. Doctors who do not want to disappoint their patients give placebos when no other medicine is warranted. Going to the doctor means you are going to take some medicine. It is the extreme reliance of allopathy on drugs for a cure that contributes to this undesirable phenomenon among the populace. Sometimes, doctors give non-specific medication to make patients feel better. The most effective drugs for these purposes are those affecting moods, such as amphetamines and tranquilizers. These kind of psychoactive drugs make patients feel better temporarily and help them forget their ailments. The repetitive use of such mood changers may cause addictions. Therefore, most doctors are disinclined to make use of psychoactive drugs. So, more and more doctors use placebos.

The term "placebo" connotes something repugnant, less serious, and unethical. But it need not be so. Some doctors and nurses give placebos to patients who seem to complain too much or exaggerate their pain. If the patient reports relief from the placebo, it is interpreted that the pain was subjective and has no objective physiological basis. A true understanding of the nature of placebos and its working on the human mind will dispel the present misgivings about placebos and will lead to the use of it in a beneficial way for building health.

In the early times, when pharmacopoeia was limited to a few herbs, the effectiveness of many medical treatments depended upon the patient's expectation of positive benefits. Medical history is replete with examples of treatments that appeared effective but later proved to have no actual curative effects any greater than the placebos could achieve. In 1979, a long history of therapies applied to reduce angina – the pain in the chest and arms caused by the decreased flow of blood to the muscles of the heart – was reviewed by Dr. Herbert Benson who reported some stunning revelations. The treatments ranged from drugs to surgeries that worked in seventy to ninety percent of the cases until a review and new research told of its ineffectiveness. They were based on the misguided belief that the treatment was working in an objective manner. With the emergence of the new findings, the effectiveness dropped to between thirty and forty percent.

Doctors and nurses know that size, color, shape and name of the placebo can influence the healing. Placebo effects can influence the outcome of a surgery. Until 1950, a surgical procedure called Internal Mammary Artery Bypass was a common treatment for heart disease. In a study, one group of patients received the true surgery and another group received a pseudo surgery. It is noted that both groups had the same degree of relief symptoms after surgery. Patients who received the pretense surgery showed a fifty percent reduction in their angina pectoris one year later when compared with the group who received the actual surgery. The consequence of the experiment resulted in stopping Internal Mammary Artery Bypass for heart problems.[3] The knowledge and belief that one's doctor is skillful and informed and knows how to take you down the road to healing helps a great deal in the process of healing. What we believe about our doctors and medical treatment will markedly affect our illness and recoveries. What you believe about your health is going to happen sooner or later.

A set of experiments described by Jerome Frank, an authority on the placebo effect, revealed how and what you believe affects what happens to you. In Frank's experiments, test patients were given one of the three substances: a mild painkiller, a harmless but ineffective placebo, and a heavy dose of morphine. When patients were given the useless placebo, but were told they were getting morphine, two-thirds of them reported that their pains disappeared. When patients were given morphine but were told they were getting a mild painkiller, over half of them said they still had pain. And, when patients were given a harmless placebo that caused headaches in previous experiments, three-quarters of them developed headaches.[4] In another experiment, when doctors administered a placebo under the impression that it was morphine, its effect on the patient increased. The experiment was then reversed. When doctors thought that the drug they administered was a placebo when, in fact, they were administering morphine, its effect on the patients diminished. Could it be that doctors can subconsciously transfer to the patient their expectation of how the drug could affect the patient? This has a wider implication when a caregiver's attitude and belief are transferred to the patient. Caregivers can be a catalyst in healing, as is the doctor.

As we have noted earlier, healing is from within. It is not doctors or medicine that heal; the body heals itself if provided with the right conditions. Our human system is wired to build health and seek healing. Our mind has powers at our disposal to use for better health. To tap our mind powers, we have to look beyond the duality of the mind and body as separate units. Our mind is present all through our body, through our brain and nervous system. The extraordinarily complex brain and nervous system assess every input in our body, such as images, thoughts, beliefs and directives, and literally reconstitutes itself and acts upon the new reconstruction. It is willing to take on any data you feed it. Your brain does not distinguish external reality from the internal. This is why when you have a bad dream and are literally frightened and scream, it causes all physiological changes of increased heart rate and blood pressure and the rush of adrenaline to the concerned organs that need to be activated.

In 1979, at Princeton University, Robert G. Jahn established a research program to explore the role of consciousness in the establishment of physical reality. After numerous controlled experiments, Jahn and his associates published their findings stating that the mind can and does directly affect physical reality. If we are deeply aware that our minds play a decisive role in constructing the physical reality, we can choose to live more creatively to enhance our health.[5] Since mind/body interactions are real and capable of creating new physical realities, medicine should take advantage of this connection to heal people. It need not be considered as trickery. Although placebos are inert substances, they work as instruments to invoke certain mind powers to effect cure. Placebos have relieved severe post-operative pain, induced sleep, and brought remission in both symptoms and objective signs of chronic diseases. Rejection of warts and the removal of abnormal growths have been effected through placebos. As every drug does not affect everyone equally, we do not expect uniform results in the administration of placebos. Healing through drug administration is oftentimes partial, and the problem may recur over the course of time. That does not tell us the drug is impotent. Belief-healing elicited through placebos is sometimes stronger and more effective than that of drug-induced healing. It is simply incorrect to think placebo responses are mild and short lasting.

The strength of placebo responses can be of any magnitude. According to medical theory, an antibiotic cannot cure a viral sore throat. But, frequently, it is administered and many are cured. Dr. Andrew Weil speaks of "Active Placebos." It is a contradiction in terms, but it is an extremely useful concept.[6] Insertion of an acupuncture needle causes pain and other sensations. By that alone, it may elicit favorable placebo responses independent of, or in combination with, any direct beneficial effect it may have on illness. Similarly, an allopathic injection can easily function as an active placebo because the patient feels it and likely believes in its curative powers. Injections are powerful, not just because they go directly into the bloodstream and targeted organs, but by those special sensations elicited, the emotional acuity, and focus given to the action, which are all helpful. Besides, most people have a belief that injections are more powerful than pills. Studies have revealed that inactive placebos work better when they taste bitter, are expensive, or eye-catching in their very shape and color. Bitter and expensive pills fit the patient's drug conceptualizations and, thus, are more convincing.

Any drug administered to patients can produce direct effects of that medicine, as well as active placebo responses, because of the belief in the drug and belief in the doctor. So, the favorable outcome of any medical intervention is the result of three factors: 1) efficacy of the medical treatment; 2) the belief system of the patient; and 3) the beliefs of the physician. The boundaries of these three factors are not easily discernible nor can they be measured. This is not a sufficient reason to overlook elements that have a much more far-reaching impact on health. Even the double-blind studies, employed to bring out the objective effect of a medicine, do not give any guarantee that something is directly the result of a medicine. There is no practical way to eliminate all elements of belief entered into the therapeutic milieu when a patient is treated. No one can draw sharp lines between mind-mediated responses and the direct effects of a drug on the body. Since there is no dichotomy between mind and body, they always interact and impinge upon each other.

Practitioners of different therapies apply methods they believe to be useful. They have some personally convincing experiences and theories in the realm. So, they are enthusiastic in the administration of their therapies. This enthusiasm and faith is contagious, and it is radiated to the patients consciously and subconsciously. The methods they use directly cause changes in some patients; sometimes the change is explainable, sometimes not. In most cases, all alternative therapies produce some beneficial results on account of the belief system as is in the case of allopathy that we have just noted. Any direct beneficial impact of a treatment can always be boosted by an additional indirect effect – a placebo effect, which is nothing other than the belief's effect.

It is shown that new drugs most often produce favorable results when they first hit the market. When the interest in the medicine is great with the doctors and the patients, remarkable results have been brought forth and it is viewed as a bright light. As time goes by, many of the drugs work less effectively. Then, some new research comes along that indicates the drug has some side effects hitherto unnoticed. Soon, the drug's efficacy will be reduced in half. The drug has not changed, but the belief in the drug has. Suddenly, the drug is seen in a dim light, and it does not look very impressive. Even with good drugs, the "field" that receives them depends on the mind-set of the person, and this produces crucial variables. People who use marijuana have shown astounding variations in response. To some, it is a stimulative; to others, it is a sedative; and, again, to some, it is an aid to sleep, while others may remain awake. There is no uniformity in reactions. That means it is not the intrinsic quality of the marijuana that sets the response but the field. The conclusion is that the pharmacological effect of marijuana is not as great as we imagine. The problems people have with narcotics are strongly influenced by the expectation and the field.

If the sensations and feelings one experiences after the administration of a drug, or any therapeutic principle, are interpreted by the mind positively, it helps to bring about a cure rapidly. Therefore, more active drugs will work more indirectly through the mind.[7] A drug that produces soreness, nausea, dizziness, and bowel discomfort is capable of bringing the mind into the action. Any surgery, in addition to its direct effect, is capable of bringing the mind into action. Allopathy is able to bring a mind-mediated healing to its patients more than therapeutic systems because of the widespread faith in technology and the relatively traumatic procedures they employ to effect physical changes that mobilize a mind-mediated healing. The point is that any system of treatment can cure people, irrespective of what direct effect the therapeutic principle makes, provided it can bring the mind into action as an indirect result of the therapeutics. Even procedures based on ridiculous theories can cure people if they work as active placebos. Much of the drugs and procedures of allopathy owe most of their value to the powers of the mind, whether one agrees with it or not. It is ironic that it is the immaterial mind that helps the materialistic medicine. There is nothing unethical in viewing placebos as a valid means of activating the mind mechanism towards a cure. Placebos can be employed creatively with good intent and enthusiasm, dropping the ambivalence and hesitation, which is now widespread.

No therapeutic system will be willing to accept that its therapeutics is less effective and that it depends on mind-mediated healing more than direct action of the therapeutic principle. Consequently, innocuous means of healing modalities are overlooked. Andrew Weil, MD, puts it in the right perspective: "Healing is an innate, latent capacity of the mind/body, waiting to be released or unblocked by methods that directly give sick people a hand in overcoming illness but succeed only if the beliefs of both patients and practitioners interact productively with them."[8] We should really attribute the success of many medical treatments to the inherent healing power within everyone.

Reconstitute Your Computer

It is estimated that more than fifty percent of the patients who visit a clinic do not have any verifiable symptoms. But, they complain about real problems they experience. Health problems, which do not have any external cause, are more likely to come from within. One cannot heal a health problem that originates from within by relying on a therapeutic system that focuses on externals. External tools and devices are good for that which comes from the external environment and stimuli. Most health problems do have a source in the internal mechanism of humans. Earlier, we have seen the human interconnectedness of the body, mind, and spirit. Though the spirit and mind have their own properties, generally, they are expressed through our body system. That is why we say humans are spirit incarnated in the body. In this life, the body is the vehicle for the expression of mind and the spirit. The most vital organ of the body is the brain, which is responsible for the quality of life. Whatever happens in the body is easily discernible from what happens in the brain. Ideas, beliefs, values, and expectations are associated with the brain and its integrity. It is the brain that translates these qualities into physiological realities.

Our knowledge and understanding of the brain is still on the primitive level. The brain, a three-pound hemisphere made of a gelatin-like substance, remains largely mysterious. Every new discovery about the brain only tells us how much more we do not know about this supercomputer. Not even our universe with its countless billions of galaxies presents a greater wonder than the human brain. It makes possible perceptions and new perspectives. Many talk about the capabilities of some mega computers, but no computer can match the potential capability of the human brain. Without causing a traffic jam or major breakdown, the brain is sending, receiving, and processing millions of messages per day. Purpose, goals, determination, self-affirmation and self-acceptance are not mere mental states. They have electrochemical connections that play a role in the entire economy of the total human organism. Now we know this much about our health: movement, intuition, memory, thoughts, and intelligence all can be traced to the brain and its specialized neurons and neurotransmitters. Each neuron comes with stringy extensions on the ends called axons and dendrites. The axons transmit messages to other nerve cells while the dendrites receive input from other axons. The brain is comprised of one hundred billion neurons or nerve cells. These microscopic nerve cells are astonishing communicators constantly passing millions of messages for the optimum function of the body. Bundled together in groups, they control and regulate different functions in the body. They act like a switchboard with an immense number of messages registered, transferred, connected, and interpreted simultaneously.

Nerve cells are so well connected that they can make a trillion connections at a given time. Messages are delivered to axons by means of a chemical courier called neurotransmitters. Axons emit chemicals at synapses, the junctures between dendrites and their neighboring nerve cells, axons. Neurotransmitters are crucial players in the orderly function of the brain; its shortage or excess will cause an imbalance in the system. Adrenalin is a neurotransmitter that stimulates heart-beating in response to a perceived threat of fight or flight. More than fifty different neurotransmitters have been identified so far, but what is most striking is that the brain retains a memory of the nerve cell activations and interactions. The brain responds to messages from the environment, the body, and the brain itself. An image or representation of every incident-taking place in relation to your body is recorded forever with all its details – emotional value, survival meaning, physical impact, etc. The brain tends to process, register, transmit, interpret, and retain memory in the same fashion whether the stimuli is from within or without. This is why suggestions, belief systems, and visualization all work to effect healing. An image is formed when a certain constellation of nerve cells is activated. To recall an image, the brain reconstructs the constellation of activity that first occurred. Patterns of activation are stored and remembered. This memory is pulled out in a similar situation. The pattern of brain activity that pulls out the associated image is called neurosignatures. All our life events and emotions have neurosignatures – shorthand notations that the brain stores and recalls.[9]

Events that have high emotional and survival value enter into the brain within no time – without waiting for our conscious processing. Your input is very minimal in such circumstances. Our brains are wired for certain instinctual behavior patterns and behaviors. This is part of the hardwiring, which we cannot change. When we receive a diagnosis or a subsequent treatment modality, our brain adds a value to it by its own nature. But, this is not something irrevocably fixed. By your conscious processing of the incident, you can add personal meaning to it and, thereby, can reconfigure and reconstitute new images and representations.

We have two different kinds of intelligence – intellectual and emotional; they express activity of different parts of the brain. The intellect is based on the neocortex, the more recently evolved part in the evolution of the human brain.[10] The emotional centers are lower in the brain – the subcortex. The neocortex and subcortex work in concert with each other; if not, it will affect the total well-being of the person. The subcortex acts as the brain's alarm. The subcortex overrides prefrontal areas of the brain in times of emergency, and a surge of emotions suspends the prefrontal circuitry. This is the hardwiring area of the brain. Since survival needs always take precedence in states of anxiety, fear, and agitation, the neocortex – where our self-regulating mechanism resides – is overridden and put out of use temporarily. Our ability to think and act in the right manner suffers. But, we can regain our self-regulating competencies by putting the neocortex back into work. Based on our beliefs, motives, values, and attitudes, the brain will begin to produce different chemicals. When one is challenged and motivated by a new outlook and vision of life, it produces a new set of neurosignatures.

Neuroscientists have documented the fact that the brain can design new patterns, new combinations of nerve cells, and neurotransmitters in response to new input. Because of the new learning, individual neurons will change, as well as the pattern of signals it sends. The ability to change the brain's new wiring to grow new neural connections has been demonstrated in experiments. In one of the experiments conducted by the *National Institute of Mental Health*, the researchers had the subjects perform a simple motor task, a finger-tapping exercise, and identified the parts of the brain involved in this task by taking an MRI (magnetic resonance imaging) brain scan. The subjects then practiced finger-tapping daily for a period of four weeks, gradually becoming more efficient and expert at it. At the end of the four weeks, the brain scan was repeated and showed that the area of the brain involved in the task had expanded, indicating that the regular practice and repetition of the task had recruited new nerve cells and changed the neural connections that had originally been involved in the task.

The brain is malleable and changes constantly, making new neurosignatures based on the new input. The brain is constantly at work recruiting new nerve cells and their activating patterns. The brain is its own artist, chemist, and engineer, constantly remaking and reconstituting itself. Scientists believe that repetition of a task brings about frequent convening of particular like-minded nerve cells; recruits other nerve cells in the cortex; and enlarges and changes the neural connections that were initially involved. That means there is a hardwiring and softwiring in our brain. The softwiring quality of the brain helps us to learn new things, attach new values and meanings to our actions, and thereby change the neurosignatures that control wellness and healing.

Because of the plasticity of the brain, we can change bad habits. We can give a new set of instructions to the brain by invoking positive beliefs, and replace the pattern of thinking it has become accustomed to. Genetic dispositions are part of our hardwiring, which one may not change easily. But, the ability of the brain to change and reconfigure itself is a great gift of the Creator. Because of bias and preconceived notions, the total potential of our mind and brain is untapped. By mobilizing our thoughts and beliefs, we can change the manner in which the nerve cells fire and make new neurosignatures. We can markedly control brain activity to promote our health and well-being by affirmations, visualization, yoga, meditation, hypnosis, and biofeedback, to name a few. These are all mind-mediated healing methods that we will read more about in the next chapter.

5

Mind-Based Healing Modalities

Researchers claim that sixty to seventy percent of hospital visits have no obvious external reason. We noted earlier, people are sick often not from external factors but from internal factors. That which originates from within has to be treated accordingly. Therapeutic principles that rely on external factors alone cannot bring about healing to people who do not have verifiable symptoms. Centuries ago Hippocrates said, "The mind is a great healer." In examining our belief system and its potential to heal, we have a profile of mind-related healing. It is not a new teaching that our minds play a major role in keeping health and well-being. Modern medicine does not give due respect to the role of the mind in restoring health and wellness. The effects on the human mechanism and its function are no longer a subject of debate. Relaxation programs give a time-out for the strained and overworked mechanism to restore itself and recuperate. The average person, as well as the medical profession, has increasingly realized now, how much the mind and physical body are intertwined.

Stress and Its Repercussions

Today, large numbers of people are suffering from stress-related problems. Stress is a physiological and psychological arousal or excitement generated to cope with the demands of the person. Our nervous system plays a crucial role in stress-related crises. A part of the nervous system, called the *autonomic nervous system,* controls our body's response to stress. It has two opposing systems; namely, the *sympathetic nervous system* (SNS = emergency system) and the *parasympathetic nervous system* (PNS = maintenance system). The SNS prepares our body by shutting down the maintenance activities of the body and collects all of its resources to deal with the immediate crisis: a fight-or-flight response. Once we have evaded the crisis, the body slows down and the PNS takes over, slowing down the heart rate, blood pressure and resuming the maintenance of the body. If there is no termination of the real or imaginary danger, one part of our system is overworked, and the other part is undercared for and, thus, goes unrepaired. In stress, the body is not able to adjust to its usual maintenance and repair mode. One system continuously works itself and burns out in the process. Therefore, stress can be defined as anything that draws attention away from the body's maintenance.

The body is not made to function with a high level of arousal for long periods of time. The organ system begins to break down with the weakest part going first. Sometimes, people have little awareness about their level of stress. Stress can be from the external environment, such as accidents, death, divorce, chronic illness, etc. It also can be from within because of someone's values, beliefs, ambitions, dreams, expectations, and frustrations related with family, career, love, etc. Whatever the external trigger may be, stress takes a heavy toll. During crisis, our body produces adrenaline, epinephrine, and other chemicals that heighten our senses and quicken our actions. In times of an emergency, stress is good; one receives extraordinary energy to accomplish the things that might otherwise be impossible. In an emergency mode, cortisol is pumped into the blood in high volume. The overall impact of cortisol is to energize the person for a fight-or-flight response. It is actualized by dulling other subtle functions of the mind. Cortisol steals energy from the working memory and transfers it to the senses. Information is not processed properly. As a result of this condition, the functioning mode is more primitive. Under stress, non-emergency functions are shut off. As endocrine glands secrete cortisol into the blood, wartime alertness is produced. The autonomous nervous system prepares the body for emergencies by conserving energy and directing it to the vital organs and their functions. Constricting small arteries at the skin level makes more blood available to the vital organs. A continued state of emergency leaves the concerned organs worn and torn. The threat may be real or imaginary, but it does not affect the mechanics.

Chronically elevated levels of cortisol are known to change the behavior of certain organs. The arteries begin to get stiff and hardened, commonly known as arteriosclerosis. Chronically elevated cortisol has been related to cancer. If stress is not handled or addressed properly, excessive production of cortisol is the result. As long as you are in a state of fear, stress, or panic, cortisol secretion continues and more and more immune cells and molecules are put up against possible threat. Since this threat is mostly imaginary, there are no actual enemies to fight, and finally the excessive antibodies turn against one's own body. The result is an autoimmune disease such as arthritis, lupus, or vasculitis. We know that any system has only a given amount of energy to be used. If you use it all at one time, you may not have enough for famine time. The body cannot produce cortisol and immune cells endlessly; the body minerals will exhaust themselves in the course of time. When the cortisol level goes down, because of the lack of stimulation, you feel depressed. The exhaustion of fighting an imaginary war leaves one defenseless in the end, having run out of all reserve ammunition. Stress, in the end, suppresses the immune system. Your body then becomes defenseless against microbes and infectious diseases. When laboratory rats were put under constant stress, cortisol and other related hormones reached toxic levels, actually poisoning and killing neurons.[1] Continued stress can weaken the memory, too.

Stress is the result of any perceived threat. The threat may be real or imaginary. Irrespective of its nature, the body begins to equip itself to fight. If the threat or crisis is imaginary, there is no object to act upon, so the activated mechanisms that fight turn against the body itself.

Stress affects the whole system. Stress-related illnesses primarily affect the mind and, through the mind, the whole functioning of the body. These types of disorders can be cured by mind mediation. Yoga, meditation, biofeedback, hypnosis, and spirituality are some of the tools to still the agitated mind. When the mind is stilled and quieted, the body begins to follow the mind and regains the lost harmony and balance in the body functions.[2]

Our organs sometimes function as warning systems, too. Generally speaking, certain organs in the body are found more vulnerable than others in the wake of any stress. The stress can be physiological or psychological. Stress affects the weakest points in the body first: for some, it may be the throat; some, the lungs; and in others, the stomach. These vulnerable points register stress as early warning signs of an impending crisis in the system. So, learning about the weakest points and observing them for early warning signs will help you to notice illness in the early stages and improve the chances of fortifying against it.

Whenever you experience stress and anxiety, your muscles tend to contract and tighten. The autonomic nervous system controls your involuntary muscles, digestive system, breathing, heart, endocrine glands, and circulatory system. It is this autonomic system that sets off responses to outside stimuli. This is the part of the nervous system involved with feelings and emotions. We do not control it; it is autonomous in its own way. The other autonomic system – the central nervous system – is made up of the brain and the spinal cord. You have more direct control over this system. You can, at your will, make different movements in your body. The autonomous nervous system in its own way responds to given stimulus and sets off intense activity in proportion to the perceived danger. These responses are immediate; they bypass the thinking centers of the brain. Still, you can train the autonomic nervous system not to respond to the perceived stress or fear. It is the real or imaginary fear that sets off the response.

Breath to Quiet the Mind

By practicing relaxation therapies, you can keep the autonomic system from placing stress on the heart, muscles, and circulatory system. Learning to relax the muscles is critical in quieting the autonomic nervous system.[3] If you keep your muscles relaxed, you will hold back the stress response. It seems that man's brain has created more than his nervous system can handle. The increased competitive tempo is contrary to nature's need for mental recuperation through tranquility and physical relaxation.[4] Relaxation exercises are a powerful tool for controlling stress and should not be underestimated.

Proper breathing nourishes the whole human organism. It can regulate moods and emotions.

Proper breathing involves proper expansion of the lungs in a systemic fashion. Learning how to breathe and working consciously with breath is simple, safe, and an inexpensive way of promoting health. The first step in proper breathing is diaphragmatic breathing. Using your diaphragm – the large muscles under your rib cage – will help to pull the air deep into your body. Breathing only in your chest is stressful breathing, while diaphragmatic breathing is relaxation breathing. Since breath is basic to human life, controlling and balancing it can order and influence the health outcome. In the yoga system, *pranayama* is the primary tool in bringing discipline to life and harmony to the system. *Prana* means 'breath' in Sanskrit. It is a controlled and rhythmic breathing. *Pranayama* can silence our mind effortlessly and help us let go of any persistent worries. Chest breathing is common when we are under stress. Breathing becomes shallow, and we do not get the needed oxygen that, in turn, leads to further stress. By focusing on breath and by simply being aware of our breathing rhythms and patterns, we can stay in the present moment. Maintaining awareness of breath keeps one constantly in the present and, thereby, the body will be relieved from the stressful patterns.

The practice of sitting and listening to and watching one's breath is a primary meditation practice in all schools of Buddhism. Listening to one's breath helps one to connect to the present moment and understand the nature of the mind. Some of the major steps you can take to practice rhythmic breathing are:

- Sit in a comfortable posture to observe or listen to your breath.
- Close your eyes gently to avoid disturbances from your surroundings.

  (When you close your eyes, practically speaking, the world is shut off, so that you can easily focus on the interior world.)
- Become aware of your breathing, its rhythm, and the rise and fall of your abdomen.
- Practice this watching or listening three to four minutes.
- Focus your inward gaze to your heart.
- Make an intention that you are quieting the mind by this act.
- Inhale deeply in a slow and gentle fashion.
- Hold your breath for five seconds and start slowly to exhale.
- On your exhalation, imagine that you are collecting up and sending out all your worries and concerns.
- Within ten minutes, you will feel relaxed, your mind empty and your worries drained.

You can practice slightly different progressive methods of relaxation. Quieting your mind is your supreme vacation and vocation.

- In a peaceful surrounding, take a comfortable posture and watch your breathing as you did it previously.
- Once you are focused on your breathing, direct your breathing into certain areas of your body, which allows your muscles to relax more readily.

- Inhale deeply into that part of the body you want to relax. Don't worry if it does not work immediately; just keep doing it. Soon you will realize it is working.
- You can progressively relax yourself in this manner from your toes to your head. Breathe into your feet, ankles, knees, thighs, buttock, chest, stomach, and so on and so forth. As you direct your breath into each area, feel that the new energy you pumped into the body by your breathing softens and energizes the organs and whole system.

When you are thoroughly focused, you can do the second phase of the relaxation. Each time you find your mind wandering, bring attention back to your breath. Do not attach any value to your performance and accomplishment level.

- Now, focus your mind on your feet, taking a deep inhalation; imagine that you are inhaling and exhaling through your feet rather than your nostrils.
- Keep doing this inhalation and exhalation exercise, gradually moving upward through all body parts. This technique will relax your body and quiet your mind.

Bastrika is another breathing technique I find very useful to release tension and stress. The Sanskrit word refers to a device that can produce a stream of air through a narrow door when pressed forcefully. Bring these mechanics to your breathing. Air is forcefully inhaled and exhaled similar to the blasting of air through a furnace. Although it is an active breathing technique, it has a calming effect on the mind. This is to be done in a straight-seated position, unlike other ones that use any comfortable position.

- Sit comfortably keeping your spine as straight as possible.
- Focus on your breath for two minutes and relax.
- Close your hands into a fist; fold your forearm parallel to your upper arm.
- Take a normal inhalation and exhalation.
- Extend your hands over your head, taking a large, forceful inhalation and opening your palms.
- Forcefully exhale, closing your arms back to the starting position.
- Repeat 15 to 20 times. You may rest in between, if you desire, for a few seconds or minutes.

Short breaths and shallow breaths upset the system's functioning. Shortness of breath is implicated in sleep disturbances, migraines, epileptic seizures, and heart problems. People who begin to breathe properly become less irritable and get along better with others. It is amazing how our quality of life can be enhanced by a simple means we can easily master.

We know that breath is basic to life. If breath is basic to human life, by controlling and balancing it, you can control and balance other functions of human life naturally.

Proper rhythm and balance in the basic substance of life are capable of bringing the same qualities throughout the system. Focusing on breath has an extraordinary power to connect us to the present. Most of our tensions and worries arise from ruminating over the past or future. Breath is something that happens moment by moment in the present. Awareness of breath keeps you connected to the present.

Meditation

Meditation is another powerful tool to relax the tone of autonomic nerves and, thereby, lower blood pressure and relieve stress on the heart, stomach, and intestines. The word for meditation in Sanskrit is *Dhyana,* which translated is 'prolonged one-pointed attention.' In Latin, the root word is *mederi,* which means 'remedy'. Put each of the word meanings together, and we arrive at a better understanding of the richness of this relaxation response. Prolonged one-pointed attention of the mind on anything positive is a remedy unto itself. In traditional meditation, a prolonged one-pointed attention is paid to an idea, a prayer, a mantra, or to your breath. By doing this, we refocus our mind from its usual thoughts of reviewing the past or planning the future to the present moment. It ultimately results in a calm and quiet mind attuned to the body. Meditation practiced well has therapeutic as well as spiritual benefits. It is the antidote for physical, mental, and emotional stress. It can lift one to the spiritual realm as well as to mystical experiences. Without attaining harmony with one's physical and emotional life, no spiritual growth and experience can be expected. So, in many religious traditions, calming the mind and attaining harmony in the system was, and is, a first step in the spiritual life. Medical science and therapists, with their characteristic reductionist tendency, took meditation for its therapeutic purpose alone. Nevertheless, by quieting one's mind through meditation, one becomes more and more aware of the nature of one's mind and its connection to the cosmos and to the Universal Mind. Those who have a spiritual interest can go deeper and can experience much more in a state of altered consciousness. Via meditation, one is able to discover and realize the Divine in oneself; as the result of that, perfect peace, joy, and a sense of fulfillment are attained. On a physiological level, meditation normalizes many of the body's functions by:

- Calming and stabilizing the nervous system
- Decreasing cortisol, the primary stress hormone
- Reducing muscle tension
- Normalizing blood pressure and serum cholesterol
- Increasing serotonin, the neurotransmitter often associated with happiness
- Reducing mental fatigue and irritability; and refreshing the self

When we meditate, we consciously guide our mental activity to a deeper level of functioning: a level where more of our mind's resources can be accessed. Research demonstrates that relaxation, without an inward mental focus, simply does not produce the same state of consciousness as meditation. Relaxation simply means relaxing our tensed muscles, whereas meditation involves relaxing mind and body in a deeper way. With the conscious mind only accounting for ten percent of our mental activity, meditation is the option to access the other ninety percent. As we quiet our mind and move to an internal silence, we begin to touch upon the vast resources of our unconscious mind. Metaphysically, it is the channel through which we communicate with our higher consciousness and the infinite intelligence of the universe.

The impulse to meditate is natural to all of us because we are programmed to search and strive for harmony within our multidimensional system. Most people seek meditation to reduce stress. Along with that benefit, they will find something more wonderful: ease in which to drop negative habits, improve relationships, achieve inner joy, love, and a forgiving attitude. So, it is worth it to try meditation on many accounts. Do not get stressed about doing it perfectly. When your mind wanders, without becoming upset, come back to your focus. You can be exploratory in your own style once you are well-grounded. Think of an experience or incident when you got lost and you did not notice how quickly the time had passed. In meditation, you allow yourself to be lost, shifting your mind away from everyday disturbing and distracting thoughts and objects. Our mind machine is spinning with millions of thoughts hour after hour. Each desire and thought generates an amount of energy. Since the needed time to process the thought and its energy is not given, at the emotional level we experience a sense of restlessness and repulsion. In the quiet times of focused attention, the brain is able to wipe out the toxic and cluttered negative energy. Therefore, it is well disposed for receiving new ideas and beliefs. Cognitive restructuring is found easy in a state of relaxation.

Different religious traditions have slightly varying approaches to meditation. Basically, they are meant to calm your mind. Lao-tzu, the Chinese philosopher, said, "Silence is revelation." Silence has the power to reveal the meaning and mysteries of life. To bring silence on, one can use rhythmic breathing or any kind of breathing exercise. When the mind is settled by focusing on one's breath, it is time to use a mantra. *Mantra* is a sacred word or phrase rich in meaning and appealing to one's personality. Your mantra is a symbol of what you are looking for or what you are seeking. By paying focused attention to it, you become one with what you focus on. Your consciousness is expanded and identified with the mantra and what it symbolizes. For an easy identification with your mantra, inhale the sacred word or phrase of your mantra. Allow yourself to feel the grace and power contained in the mantra (any thought or intention is a form of energy); you are slowly inhaling, thereby assimilating the energy into your whole system. Let yourself become filled with this new mantra energy. When you slowly rise up from meditation, you will experience a sharper mind, relaxed muscles, and a positive energy for life.

Healing Meditation

There is no standardized meditation that works equally for all. One has to find out one's own model creatively and exploratively. There is no right or wrong method. According to your personality type, you may be drawn to different traditions. The steps for a simple healing meditation are as follows:

- Take a favorite meditation posture.
- Close your eyes and focus your gaze inward.
- Focus on your breath and settle your mind.
- Make the intention to increase your harmony, or to heal yourself, or expand your consciousness.
- As you enter into a deeper silence and quietness through breathing, silently say to yourself or affirm *your* mantra:

"I am in full harmony and balance".

- Attune your mantra with the inhalation so that after repetition, you do not have to verbalize it. It will automatically happen with your inhalation.
- As you go through this process, your mantra can be reduced to a minimum; now you only need two words – "***harmony and balance***".
- Gradually, you can reduce it to one word with all the meaning symbolized into one word – ***"harmony" or "balance***".

- Slowly, in your exhalation, you can also use a phrase or mantra. For example, ***"I am healed and restored".***
- Reduce that mantra, too, as you progress further in silence and quietness – "***healed and restored".*** Again, finally reduce the mantra to one word of your choice: "***healed" or "restored".***
- Spend twenty to thirty minutes in this meditation. Slowly 'wake' yourself to experience the newfound energy and harmony in your life.

Meditation is a means of self-awareness and self-knowledge. Stress and fatigue of the body and mind deprive us of our innate goodness. Practicing meditation restores us, bringing a quiet mind during and after meditation. I believe that meditation is a God-given faculty to restore and refresh us, free of cost, and without any harmful side effects, but with wholesome effects.

A significant character of any relaxation program is its ability to bring down the rate of metabolic activity. Our body is in constant need of energy to meet its various ongoing functions. The cells in our body burn nutrients with the help of oxygen and generate the energy needed for the heart, lungs, and brain that are constantly working. In our waking and active engagement times, we need more fuel; whereas when we sleep, we need less fuel. A sleeping time of between six to eight hours is necessary for all of us because this is the time our metabolic rate goes down, and the concerned system gets the needed rest to recuperate. The controlled rhythmic breathing and meditation modes slow the metabolic rate that occurs similar to the sleep state. The reaction is almost opposite of what happens in an emergency mode. In this state, every mental, emotional, and physical activity is at its highest point and requires all the systems to produce and use its maximum. People who practice relaxation methods are found to have slower frequency beta rhythms, which are associated with feelings of pleasure. Just as repeated activation of the fight-or-flight response can lead to sustained problems in the body mechanics, so too, repeated activation of relaxation practices practiced over time can mend the internal wear-and-tear brought on by stress.[5] The cumulative effects of relaxation make possible a healthy equilibrium. To the extent that any condition is caused or worsened by stress, relaxation techniques can be effective at curing or improving these conditions.

Biofeedback

Biofeedback is a mechanism that can regulate the autonomous nervous system. It lets the patient monitor the functions they wish to control. It is based on our ability to control the functions of our body by conscious decision, will, and commitment. In biofeedback training, people learn to increase blood flow to the hands by relaxing the autonomous nerves that regulate the circulatory system. This is done by paying attention to the temperature of the skin on their finger, which is converted to an audio or visual display in order to provide continuous feedback. Stress causes the heightening of arousal: an increase in the rate of the heartbeat, blood pressure, muscle tension, peripheral vascular constriction, and in most cases, rapid respiration. The underlying principle behind biofeedback is that stress and non-stress cannot exist in the human organism at the same time.[6] Individuals are helped to monitor their stress levels and, if found too high, helped to lower them by relaxation exercises then and there. Slowly, the patient learns to lower the body's functions without needing input from the biofeedback machine. Medical researchers believe that by a slow pace, one can bring a measure of control over the autonomic nervous system.

In some countries, there are preventive group programs that give training in stress management. The aim of such groups is to teach participants to recognize their own responses to stress and learn to modify their internal and external environments. Physically getting away from a stressful environment is vital. To keep stress at bay is to relax. Many relaxation techniques have been developed and perfected; most of them having their roots in Eastern spiritual traditions.

Hypnosis

Hypnosis is looked down upon to be theatrical entertainment more than a technique of scientific medicine. It is an altered state of consciousness evoked by strong suggestions. The general belief about hypnotism is that the hypnotist possesses magical powers that conquer the mind of the subject by some supernatural technique. Actually, what the hypnotist does is to help the patient relax. As we have noted earlier, in the relaxed state, one tends to receive new suggestions, ideas, and beliefs. A greater receptivity is created in our mind in the relaxed state. In this new receptive soil, the hypnotist plants strong beliefs by way of suggestions.

During hypnosis, psychosomatic changes are observable in good hypnotic subjects. Ordinarily speaking, people do not control their skin reactions to heat or cold. The nerves controlling the skin belong to the involuntary or autonomous nervous system. Some kind of circuit exists between the mind and nerves that conveys the suggestions received in a hypnotically-induced state. Therefore, the involuntary functions such as digestion, respiration, and the circulatory system they control can be influenced, and change can be effected in their functioning. They are not fully out of our control. It is noted that a calming suggestion in a crisis helps stop the gushing of blood. Authentic yoga practitioners are able to demonstrate voluntary control of the autonomous nervous system by practicing mental and physical exercises as are prescribed in the yoga system. You do not need a hypnotist to draw upon hypnotic benefits. Self-hypnosis can be practiced by learning to relax and giving suggestions to your mind in the relaxed state.

Advertisers of commercial products and services make use of the principles of hypnosis.[7] As we sit relaxed before the TV, home movie theater, or other such entertainment location, we are easily absorbed by the suggestions directed at us. During such periods, we are extremely vulnerable because we are in a relaxed state and our brain waves have changed to *alpha*. Generally, in most TV shows, we see the same advertisements repeated during every commercial break. Repetition enforces suggestion and finally enforces behavior into the reflexes of the nervous system. Each time an experience is repeated by imagining, visualizing, or firmly believing in something, a marking is made on the cortex of the brain. By repetition, it is engraved in the brain to experience it later in similar situations. One can reinforce positive experiences and engrave them in the consciousness by doing it in a state of relaxation more than by any other means.

What is vital in hypnosis is that when you are in this receptive relaxed mode, repetition slowly leads to a conditioning. Our brain absorbs information through our senses. The output of the mind will be in accordance with the input. Hypnosis is the art of positive suggestion given in an optimum environment. You do not need a hypnotist to practice it; self-hypnosis is equally workable to reverse negative health conditions and habits.

Visualization

Any change of focus in attention gives signals of change in the body, especially when it is a change from toxic negative thoughts and images. Visualization is based on the principle that if you hold on to an image or picture in your mind long enough, it will be translated to physical reality as signified by the imagery. American psychologist and philosopher William James remarked that we think in terms of pictures just as we dream in pictures. Words are symbols enabling us to communicate or describe those pictures. If you can learn to hold those pictures long enough without letting them weaken, you will convert those pictures into reality.[8] The mind-body connection is stronger than most of us imagine. Many studies testify to the fact that visualization and imagery create and have a positive effect on the body. Getting started with visualization and imagery is simple. You do not need any extra or special equipment. It is all within you – in your mind.

- Assume a comfortable posture and relax by focusing on your breath.
- Visually create a healing image.
- Integrate both emotions and image.
- Add physical sensations such as feeling relieved from pain or discomfort, and experience a pleasantness or cooling effect on the concerned spots as you imagine and hold the imagery lively in your mind.
- For example, if you have asthma, picture your bronchial tubes opening in a slow and steady fashion as some powerful energy current is passing through them. Consequently, you begin to feel some sensations differently.
- Let go of the picture and hold the feeling.
- Details are critical in the use of imagery.

- Make your visualization experiential.
- Do it for ten minutes daily. After doing it for a few days, you need not set apart a time and space to do it; it becomes natural to catch these imageries at any time you will it. Then, you will be able to do it many times a day by keeping a mindfulness without any effort.

The works of Jeanne Achterberg and Frank Lowlis, pioneers in the clinical use of imagery, have amazing things to say. Working with one hundred twenty-six cancer patients, they demonstrated that future growth or remission of cancer was directly related to the specificity, vividness, strength, and clarity of their mental imagery.

Visualization is not a new technique. Everybody uses it in everyday life. We tend to picturize all our actions and make plans beforehand. Anything we plan and design first occurs in our mind by means of mental imageries and pictures. We constantly visualize how to perform a task, how to dress for an occasion, or how to play a game. We have been using our mind to create realities for centuries.[9] In visualization, you do it in a specialized fashion to create a definite result. It is impossible for the brain to feel the difference between an imagined experience and a real experience. For this reason, when we imagine something to be true, a certain part of the brain accepts this image as true and acts upon that image.

People often complain that they tried, and the image did not materialize as they pictured it. This may be due to many reasons. The premise of visualization is that the body responds to what the mind tells it to do because of its intimate connection with the body. The mind feeds information and messages to the body by means of symbols, beliefs, images, etc. A firm conviction of the mind-body connection, and the willingness of the mind to help us in need, must be at the backdrop of the work.

Hold on to an image or picture in your mind long enough in a relaxed state, and it will be translated to physical reality.

It is important to realize that the effects of visualization are not as readily obvious as the effects of drug therapy. The more you know about the basic functions of the body and their affected parts and the step-by-step healing process, the more you will be able to instruct the body in a better way. The success rate depends upon how well we employ our mental and emotional energies in a targeted manner. Clarity in the imagery and the power of concentration all vary from individual to individual. Remember, no drug therapy works equally for all. In any given situation, many factors are at play. This is true of any kind of healing modality. To be effective, all mind-related healing models might start with the guidance of a therapist or someone who has skill in the area. When someone guides us, better focusing and clarity may be achieved. No one can master any art overnight. It takes time to change from old patterns to new.

Wayne Dyer, speaking on visualization, refers to four *R's* that can make visualization an effective tool. The first *R* stands for what you *Really Wish.* The second R is for what you *Really Desire.* The third R is for what you *Really Intend.* And the fourth R stands for what you feel *Really Passionate About.* So it is all about "What you *Really, Really, Really, Really* want, you will get."[10] Keep the passion for your cause burning within you. If you visualize intensely for a half-hour, and the rest of the day is plagued by doubts, anxieties, negative thoughts and images, you are neutralizing the effect by holding negative images and pictures for a longer period of time. When we worry about illness, failure, loss, etc., we are automatically making mental pictures accordingly and tend to make them a reality. Through images and pictures, we give a blueprint to our mind to translate it to a physical reality within us. Norman Vincent Peale, in his very popular book *Positive Imaging,* states that all the ingredients of success are right inside of you if you will just turn your thinking around.

The most effective way the will of an individual can be exercised is not directly, but indirectly, through images. In the last twenty-five years, there has been a wealth of significant research on the dynamic effects of images on our personal development and growth. These images are not simple pictures in our imagination, but deep-seated energy patterns that can move and direct our lives.

Western medicine has not always considered the value of mind power in the treatment of diseases. Children and women are better candidates for visualization. Children have less preconceived notions that block the work; women are generally much more open with anything that has to do with the psychological aspect of illness. Men are more oriented to a technological fix and letting someone else do it for them. With practice, anyone can make visualization work for himself, if sufficiently motivated.

Affirmations

The power of positive thinking and affirmation can hardly be overlooked. All of what we discussed regarding other relaxation techniques are applicable here, too. By simply allowing yourself to hold an idea or thought, you are creating a field of energy that tends to attract a similar thought or idea. If you constantly think of illness, you are likely to attract more of the energy that may make you ill. When someone is negative, insecure, angry and anxious, they will be attracting the very same experiences that they wish to avoid. This is because they are constantly sending out signals that affect themselves negatively. If they send out positive signals, they will go forward and collect the same kind of experiences. Incredible! There is a lot of truth in it. '*Casual*' thoughts of affirmation and '*casual*' positive thoughts may not help greatly. However, '*positive*' thoughts and '*positive*' affirmations can speed up your recovery and the healing process. They have a power to release beneficial hormones in the body to heal itself. Several sample affirmations are listed below, namely:

- I choose health and happiness
- Abundant health is flowing to me
- I begin to enjoy health for all times
- Day by day I am restored and improved
- I receive health and blessings freely
- The Transcendent, Universal Mind, freely bestows all I need

Affirmations are positive thoughts and statements. Continuous positive thoughts and statements will work almost magically. When you make an affirmation, you should really believe that it will work. That which you do not fully believe with all the fiber of your being will not work effectively for you. Affirmations are to be made in the present tense. They can be practiced everywhere, anywhere, silently or aloud. I would ask my clients to write down their affirmations and speak them loudly outdoors a few times a day, as well as before a mirror. And I could see it working. Constantly used affirmations become beliefs. We already discussed how beliefs work. The need for continuous positive thinking and affirmation is made necessary by the fact that there is a continuous inner dialogue within our mind that is negative and constricting. The mind always needs something in which to be engaged. That is the nature of the mind: it abhors a vacuum. Therefore, if you do not give something new and reinforce it to the mind by repetition, the mind will begin to toss around old ideas, concepts, and beliefs. With positive thoughts and affirmations, you are feeding your mind with beneficial thoughts and images. If something is worth saying and affirming, it is worth repeating many times, especially when it can promote healthy life. Affirmation used in conjunction with conventional, medical, or other alternative therapies will speed up the healing process.

Preoccupation with health is a kind of affirmation of one's sickness. However, it will produce counter results. The fear of illness, real or imaginary, paralyzes the mind-body powers needed for healing. As we know, the mind does not distinguish the difference between real and unreal. It is not equipped to do so. Your mind will yield the results irrespective of the reality of your thoughts. Simply stated, people who fear diseases are more likely to get a disease. Feeding the mind with negative thoughts and expectations has a toxic effect. When the mind is free of pressures and worries, it brings better results to the whole system. Couples, who have been childless for years, after they finally give up their efforts and adopt a child, often find all of a sudden to be conceiving the baby they longed for. This can happen when the preoccupation and pressures have been lifted.

Intimacy, Compassion, and Love

Everyone wishes to have good health, a long life, peace of mind, happiness, and joy. There is scientific evidence that these things can be enhanced by feelings of love, compassion, and intimacy. Compassionate people reveal a sense of abandonment so that when they sleep, they can relax and let go. Being suspicious of other people and their activities and movements makes you tense. Compassion and love make you free, says the great Tibetan spiritual leader Dalai Lama. It helps you to trust others. It helps one to step up the immunoglobulin and such antibodies that fight against infections and diseases. People who do works of charity out of true compassion and love have more immunity against disease than other people who work in the same environment with different motives.

In one well-known experiment, David McClelland, a psychologist at Harvard University, showed a group of students a film of Mother Teresa working among the poor of Calcutta. The film stimulated in the students feelings of love and compassion. Most of them expressed a desire to work among the poor. When the saliva of these students was tested, an increase in antibodies was found. Another study conducted by the University of Michigan found that by doing regular volunteer work, interacting with others in a calm and compassionate way, life expectancy and overall vitality of the individual increases dramatically. Compassionate love promotes a positive state of mind, thereby greatly enhancing physical health, which has been documented in a number of cases.

People who volunteer to help other people out of compassion develop a distinct feeling of calmness and enhanced self-worth following the activity. Caring behaviors provide an interaction that is emotionally nourishing. By developing compassion and altruism, one can promote not only the well-being of others, but of oneself, too. F.W.H. Myers, a great parapsychologist, suggests that love, compassion, and empathy somehow make it possible for the mind to transcend the limitations of the body. He was struck by the fact that people who are telepathic with each other (individuals who could share thoughts at great distances) were frequently connected emotionally with each other deeply and lovingly. Empathy and love bond people in a mysterious way. Compassionate love connects distant organisms. Empathy and love form a literal bond – a resonance between living things. When empathic connections are made, feelings experienced by one individual also may be felt by another. Love is intimately related with health. It is not a mere romantic concept. Throughout history, TLC (Tender Loving Care) has been valued as an element of healing. The great advantage of love-medicine is that it has no side effects.

The awesome healing power of love is best illustrated by what happens when it is lost. People who lose their loved ones by death develop a greater range of health problems and live shorter lives after the incident.

It is no secret that unhappy, isolated, and lonely people get sick in greater numbers than people who are happy, humorous, and easy going. Recent medical research into humor and health has shown that laughter releases two important types of hormones from the brain: enkephalins and endorphins, which relieve pain, tension, and depression.

Social Support

Our lives revolve around many relationships. Human nature being social, the optimum functioning of the human takes place in the social context. We need each other in many different ways. Lack of human companionship has been linked to the depression of the human immune system. A study made on medical students found that lonelier students have lower 'natural killer' activity. Social support and a sense of belongingness, to either religious or secular groups where one is understood and valued, give great consolation and strength in times of stress. The mere loving presence of others causes our brain to produce endorphins that induce a sense of well-being. When someone enters into a community of people who share the same values and beliefs, the sense of solidarity becomes an inner strength that unleashes so many other mechanisms in the body to boost the well-being of the individual.

British psychologist John Browly wrote, "Intimate attachments to other human beings are the hub around which a person's life revolves..." From these intimate relationships and attachments, a person draws strength and enjoyment of life; and through what one contributes, one gives strength and enjoyment to others. These are matters about which current science and traditional wisdom are one. Intimacy promotes physical and psychological well-being. Medical researchers have found that people who have close relationships – people to whom they can turn for affirmation, affection, and empathy – are more likely to survive health challenges and less likely to develop diseases.

Compassionate love can produce a greater number of antibodies. A loved one's presence causes the brain to produce endorphins that promote a sense of well-being.

A study conducted in 1,000 heart patients at Duke University Medical Center found that those who lacked a spouse or close confidant were three times more likely to die within five years of diagnosis of heart disease compared to those who were married or had a close friend. Another study revealed that people who have more social support or intimate relationships have lower death rates overall and lower rates of cancer, too. Numerous studies and investigations have affirmed the fact that close relationships do promote health and overall well-being. Erich Fromm remarked, "Mankind's basic fear is the threat of being separated from other humans." He came to the view that an experience of separateness first encountered in infancy is the source of all anxiety in human life.

Good family relationships and social support are powerful elements in promoting health and healing. In the Bible's book of Genesis, after creating Adam, God said: "It is not good for man to be alone. I will make him a helper as his partner." (Genesis 2:18). The Creator of the institution of marriage was foreseeing its advantages. Many scientific studies of the health of single, married, and divorced people have proven the importance of a successful marriage being related to the physical and emotional well-being of the individuals. There are abounding studies that demonstrate the negative consequences of failed marriages and fragmented families relating to the health of the people involved. Often, people who are separated or divorced receive hospital psychiatric care nearly twenty times more frequently than married people. Divorced people are seen developing cancer at an alarming rate.[11] It is the loneliness and the increased stress related to and caused by the divorce that are directly linked to this health problem.

A problem that affects people of all ages and walks of life is loneliness. In the increasing fragmentation and disintegration of families, individuals are suffering more and more from loneliness. The root of our existence is interwoven. It cannot be separated without having the experience of hurt, pain, and stress. Humans cannot survive in isolation. Since society is becoming even more transient and less community-oriented, the social support network is at its lowest point. As people become more and more isolated and lonely, they are less able to resist infection and recover from illness. In a 1997 study published in *The Journal of the American Medical Association*, it found that people who have a great variety of social relationships were more able to resist infection with the common cold virus. The advantages of social support are far greater than a simple resistance to the cold virus. Researchers at Stanford University found that women with breast cancer who took part in support groups lived an average of eighteen months or more than patients who did not participate. It is not fully known how social support boosts the immune system, but the studies afford the possibility that social support can act as a vital component of health.

We are in a world woven with relationships and endearment. Close endearing relationships are needed for humans to grow healthily. The full potential of human nature blooms only in an atmosphere of support, understanding, and companionship. When these are lacking, lives are empty and less fulfilled. Redford B. Williams, director of behavior medicine research at Duke University in North Carolina, conducted a five-year long study of heart patients. He found that those who have neither a friend nor a spouse were three times more likely to die than people involved in strong relationships.

Psychic Healing

Psychic healers claim that they can heal others through psychic powers. They see themselves as endowed with certain powers of mind that can bring healing independent of the patient's belief. There have been gifted people throughout the decades who could make a diagnosis easily just by looking at the patients. Some had only to ask a few basic details of the patient's state of health. Psychic healing is a hot topic that draws people to opposite camps. Any model of healing not easily explicable was derided by the opposite camps and looked down upon by the so-called 'scientific' as cheats and tricksters. Self-styled guardians of science tend to ridicule any extraordinary psychic occurrences as a threat to logic and reason. One cannot deny psychic healing; for, it is possible there exists phenomena that are not understood with our present knowledge and learning. We have to admit that our knowledge is imperfect. It is ridiculous to deny something because we cannot understand it now. Telepathy, psychokinesis, precognition and clairvoyance are certain phenomena still in need of explanation. The nature of reality, as indicated by the contemporary physicists, is so much stronger than any scientists could have imagined a hundred years ago. A natural conclusion from quantum physics is that we are all representations of interrelated energy. We are primarily energy beings currently having a physical experience. Since we are primarily energy beings, or spiritual beings, we can send and receive 'thought energy'. Telepathy is mainly sending and receiving 'thought energy' from one mind to another. What we receive is affected by how we have tuned and focused our consciousness.

Through the Jungian theory of Collective Unconscious, we know that humans can draw information from sources other than the conscious mind. The vastness and depth of the mind has not yet been fully unraveled. A great deal more about the working of the mind is yet to be seen. Our collective unconscious as proposed by Jung is a storehouse of universal symbols, knowledge, and wisdom that is closed to ordinary consciousness but accessible to the unconscious mind. Some people are able to tap into these sources of wisdom and knowledge. Edgar Cayce, known as the sleeping prophet, enjoyed extraordinary psychic knowledge. He entered into a trance state and came up with diagnoses and prescriptions, which need the expertise of an MD. He could gain access to a different source of knowledge and wisdom, but once he woke up, he had no idea of what knowledge and wisdom he had conveyed. It seems that part of our mind is not restricted by time and space. Some people are able to enter into the infinite realm of the mind: sometimes by their very nature and sometimes by some of their practices.

Self-Awareness and Empowerment

There are many healing modalities coming from different traditions. But only when one stops the denial, and opens oneself up, does one set foot on the healing journey. Without empowering oneself, no true healing can take place. The first part of empowering oneself is to assume the responsibility of one's life. According to Caroline Myss, the success of any holistic tool rests on two critical points: the patient's courage to evaluate oneself honestly and the patient's ability to make choices that authentically empower the spirit.[12] Often, there is a need for new learning because a person must learn to relate his thoughts, emotions, and imagination as power tools that have the power to rebuild health. Physicians, therapists, and other health practitioners serve more in the capacity of facilitators for the healing process than as the person in charge.

If we assume the premise that illness comes from the outside by chance or fate – in the form of genes, viruses or bacteria – then we become helpless. It is this sense of helplessness that has aided the traditional medical model to survive. Once you are sick, it is not your responsibility to be cured but the doctors' with their skills. You simply receive whatever recommendation they offer in good faith. By such passivity and lack of choice, what one can receive is not health but mere palliation. We are not made better by manipulating our organs, systems, and tissues with the help of drugs and surgeries. Real health and wellness remain afar unless a person takes responsibility for healing by one's own choice and transforms his present state of consciousness.

Dr. Rudolph Ballentine, who created a unique synthesis of different healing arts, views self-awareness as the basic tool that steers one to the proper directions.[13] What the laboratory tests tell you are not sufficient. The true lab is your body. Experiments going on within the body constantly allow you to find out what suits you and what does not suit you. You are the one constantly seeing, feeling, and experiencing what is happening in your system. What creates a sense of total well-being, clarity of mind, or energy for one's tasks cannot arise from lab work, diagnosis, and drugs, but from awareness – an awareness that allows you to pick up signals and make adjustments in life. By the time you receive a diagnosis, the sickness could become irreversible, and it already might have done its damage. The awareness of one's body with its unique reactions and processes, and its symptoms and strengths, guides one to decipher the problems before the body breaks down.

If we forget our creative power to transcend our limitations, no creative power from outside will come to heal us. Denial and self-pity block creativity from within and shut off other channels to flow.[14] Once we discover that we are made or bent in a certain direction, we have to decide to go with the bend until we break, or to do everything in our power not to succumb to the disposition. There is never a good excuse to fail. The challenge is to accept the hardships, and move beyond them to find healing and wholeness. Life force or life energy visits us when we show our willingness to transcend our limitations, whatever sort it may be.

Medical science acts on the belief that there is only physical force in the universe and believes that by manipulating this force, you can restore health and wholeness. We need medical disciplines that can accommodate and acknowledge non-physical energies and forces. It is the experience of mankind that a non-physical force or some spiritual energy is active in the world of being. Health and illness are dynamic interactions of this physical and non-physical energy. Wholeness is impossible without an understanding of the spiritual energy that surrounds you and interacts with you.

6

Tips and Tools Towards Building Health

In the previous chapters, we discussed the nature of health from different conceptualizations. We closely observed the mind and its role in bringing about health and healing. The body is the vehicle through which we realize our higher purposes. The body is the temple of the spirit and its energies. He who keeps and maintains the body with the awareness of its dynamics will enjoy life, realizing the full potential of the self. Health is not a question of merely good genes and constitution, though they do play a role. We know that the body has the inherent ability to establish, maintain, and restore health. The body has a natural ability to heal itself if we remove obstacles from its path and create a healthy internal and external environment. Diet, exercise, and lifestyle can build or shatter health. The ultimate goal of any healthcare system should be prevention. The emphasis on building health has received scant attention compared to the energies and monies spent on fighting disease.

Promoting Health with Natural Therapies

Naturopathic medicine, sometimes called Naturopathy is as old as healing itself. All therapies that are exclusively natural and non-toxic can be considered part of naturopathy. These include clinical nutrition, herbal medicine, hydrotherapy, physical medicine, homeopathy, reflexology, aromatherapy and counseling. The word 'physician' is from the Greek root word meaning "nature". Hippocrates, who lived 2,400 years ago, can be considered the precursor of natural therapies. His formulation of the concept "Vis Medatrix Naturae" (the healing power of nature) is the maxim for all of these various therapies. This concept has long been the core of all indigenous medicines in almost all cultures. The earliest doctors worked with herbs, foods, water, fasting, and tissue manipulation – all gentle treatments that do not obscure the body's own healing powers. Ayurveda, a medical philosophy and herbal medicine orignating in India, existed and helped people for thousands of years before the advent of Western medicine. Hydrotherapy was used in ancient Greece and Rome. Fragrant oils and aromatherapy was in vogue in ancient Egypt.

Today's professional naturopaths make use of the latest discoveries in the field of nutrition, botanicals, homeopathy, and other natural treatments. Many of the natural therapies are complementary as they boost the healing power of the body. In this sense, they are considered complementary medicine. But, in some cases they can be the primary therapy and can be curative, especially in diseases such as ulcerative colitis, asthma, flu, allergy, obesity, chronic fatigue, etc.

All naturopaths are disinclined to use surgery and drugs unless there is grave urgency. They share certain beliefs about health and healing. Benedict Lust, who spearheaded naturopathy in the modern era, remarked: "Most people die from the effects of wrong living and drugs… Most diseases and chronic sicknesses are only aggravated by the use of medicines." Generally, all naturopaths emphasize preventive methods. Fresh air and light, good diet and water, right breathing and stretching, and herbs are some simple measures all naturopaths are likely to use in addition to their specialties. There are two schools of thought about medicine and health that are represented respectively in naturopathy and allopathy by Hygeia, the Greek goddess of health, and Asklepios, the Greek god of medicine. Medical writer and philosopher Rene Dubos states these traditions succinctly as follows: "For the worshippers of Hygeia, health is the natural order of things; a positive attribute in which men are entitled, if they govern their lives wisely. According to them, the most important function of medicine is to discover and teach the natural laws that will ensure man a healthy mind in a healthy body. More skeptical or wiser in the ways of the world, the followers of Asklepios believe that the chief role of the physician is to treat disease, to restore health by correcting any imperfections caused by accidents of birth or life."[1] The two different traditions can coexist, complementing each other without dominating each other or driving out the other. No system being perfect, there is ample room to learn from each other.

Faith in science is good and beneficial. Equally good and more beneficial is to have faith in nature and its curative powers.

There is no medicine, I believe, that works for hepatitis; only rest and diet for several months. But in a week's time, some natural herb concoction can restore the person, relieving the symptoms. This I state not as hearsay, but by having seen the specific cure in my own immediate family. People are generally more and more disenchanted with conventional orthodox medicine because of its cost, side effects, invasive nature and lengthy procedures. The early part of the twentieth century witnessed an amazing advance in drug development. It led many to think that good health can be found in the medicine chest. The growth rate of cancer, heart problems, diabetes, and AIDS all shattered humankind's illusion of the dependence on medicine.

Currently, there has been a shift in the way people think about health. People are now willing to try unconventional methods that were previously overpowered by the viewpoint of Western science and medicine's initial aura. Since the aura faded, interest in the natural methods of healing has increased all over the world from the 1980's to the present time. The medical community is slow to admit the advantages of other medicines. Many patients are attracted to the alternative or complementary medicines because of the emphasis on treating the whole person.

Ayurveda treats people by determining their mind/body type, believing that true healing depends on balancing physical, mental, and emotional influences.[2] All naturopaths claim that their treatment is directed to the underlying cause on all levels, the root cause, rather than symptomatic expressions. Good holistic practitioners will look for aspects of daily lives such as job stress, marital problems, diet, sleeping habits, etc., when determining the course of therapy. One of the principal goals of natural therapies as presented by Wolfkain, a holistic practitioner, is to help the patient take charge of his health. The whole idea is to help the patient break the cycle of dependence, to get people well, and to keep them out of the doctor's office when it is not necessary.[3] The physician's role is to facilitate, remove obstacles to health and recovery, and to support the creation of a healthy internal and external environment.

Herbal Therapy

In the past, all medicines were herbs. Primitive man discovered in the beginning of human civilization itself that plants have medicinal properties. He might have noticed it by observing animals eating certain plants and grass when they were sick in order to get well. In the course of history, humans discovered more about plants, and by a trial-and-error method, learned their potential to heal and restore. They also learned that some plants and their use could cause harm. Thus, they found plants that helped them to sleep and to stay awake, plants that cured stomachaches, and plants that soothed a bruise or cut. These primitive discoveries were systematized in India, China, Egypt, and Greece. Herbal remedies continued for centuries and were strengthened by observation and study.

Until recent decades, herbal medicine has been a rural folk phenomenon. To the urban population, it was something primitive and superstitious. Conventional medicine often handily dismissed all other medical traditions. They dismissed even the well-researched and documented advances made by those who worked in the field of natural therapies. Modern science and its knowledge of chemistry helped scientists to isolate the active ingredients from the herb and produce more potent and fast-acting medicines. Through this reductionist method, the wholesome effect of the herb is often lost.

Orthodox medicine pushed harsh treatments even when they knew that the outcome was negligible. Most cancer patients are driven to chemotherapy though there is no evidence that those methods will prolong life or relieve suffering. Because of the fear of being ridiculed or looking less scientific, many physicians avoid gentler alternatives. Knowing that orthodox medicine is good at making dramatic results, patients and families look to orthodox medicine; only when everything else fails do they look for other alternatives. The time has come to rediscover our relationship with nature and draw from its curative powers. It is reasonable to think that since nature supplies all our foods from the vegetable or herb kingdom, so should she supply all the remedies for our diseases.[4]

Plants and humans are on the same planet, sharing air, water, light, and minerals. Like humans, plants also encounter heat, cold, and wind and adjust and adapt themselves to different environments. There is a visible and invisible subtle connection that exists between humans and plants. Most plants are therapeutic in one way or another. Plants have a peculiar quality inherent to them that can draw us to the complex network of the interactional forces of nature to reorganize the lost rhythms and vibrations in our system. An unbiased student of natural science can observe certain basic organizational patterns in plants and humans. A particular plant and a specific person can share certain patterns of function. When such congruence is found, that plant can create a resonance that can be used therapeutically. The individualized medicine of homeopathy is based on this congruence and resonance. Natural medicines are made from the same living matrix that nurtures and sustains humans. Therefore, they can convey complex, natural, and informational patterns that can be used by the common system to re-program the mind and body.

To people who are in good health, herbal remedies offer opportunities for staying well. Bruises, swelling, sprains, cuts, colds, fevers, minor rashes, and burns all respond well to herbal treatments. A recovery that can be accomplished by simple, inexpensive, and less costly methods is sometimes treated with expensive, invasive, impersonal, and harmful methods of orthodox medicine, only to complicate the whole context in the end. Herbal remedies form a first-line defense against colds, flu and other infectious diseases. Unlike antibiotics, herbs can be used to treat both bacterial and viral infections. Herbal remedies sometimes work when orthodox medical treatments fail. They are great for treating urinary tract infections, digestive problems, menstrual cramps, cough, colds, allergies, fatigue, and all kinds of immune system problems. Herbs provide steady but slow, long-lasting action without any side effects. It is often our impatience and desire for convenience that drives us to synthetic drugs. Most people who do not get results with herbs make the mistake of giving up too soon. They do not wait long enough for the herb to be effective. Herbal remedies are good, but that does not imply in any sense that all remedies are absolutely safe. You must be aware that just because it is natural, it may not always be protective. Most herbal remedies are safe but a few can be dangerous, especially for people who have pre-existing health problems.

To heal is to make whole. Part of our wholeness is our connection with the plant life of the planet. In numerous ways we relate with plants. Using plants as medicine is an expression of our connection and revitalizes our participation on all levels. Reaching out for an herbal remedy is a step forward to returning to a healthful relationship in the world you inhabit.

Right Food is Right Medicine

'An apple a day keeps the doctor away.' Many may ask, 'Does it really do so?' An apple a day may be impotent to do such a task. The meaning, however, is clear. Fresh natural fruits and vegetables and such gifts of nature, if used sufficiently, can make a difference. Scientists have discovered how nutrition can stave off everything from heart disease to aging. "Let food be your medicine and medicine be your food" said Hippocrates, the father of medicine. He realized centuries ago the significance of what you eat. After depending on drugs and high-tech surgery, many are finally heeding Hippocrates. In earlier days people ate what they grew. Everybody had a small farm where they could collect whole foods high in nutrients and fiber and low in fat. Gardens served as medicine chests and their kitchens acted as pharmacies.[5]

With the arrival of the Industrial Revolution, a new way of eating and a new attitude toward food developed. Large-scale farming of feed for cattle, pigs, and chickens made meat so plentiful and cheap. High-tech processing made it available in every place and at every time. Diet, as the result of this, went from low-fat, high-fiber food to high-fat, low-fiber food. Most plant-based food systems were slowly replaced by animal sources. Simultaneously, the need for manual labor was cut down in the lives of many because machines began to work instead of human hands. As the result of the Industrial Revolution, our life environment dramatically changed. More and more people were attracted to office work that is sedentary in nature. A high caloric intake of an animal-based diet continued with less movement of the body. This all led to many diseases. Before 1900, hardening of the arteries – arteriosclerosis – was almost an unheard of thing. Now, it is one of the most prevalent problems in many developing countries, as well as under-developing countries. People started relying on the wonder drugs and paid less attention to the root causes of many diseases. Diet is believed to play a crucial role in approximately thirty percent of cancers. Gary Null, who has authored many books on health building, remarked: "We are ultra liberal in creating diseases and radically conservative in the areas of preventing and treating."[6]

Many people are unaware of the problems caused by high-fat food. Nutritionists say that ideally fat should comprise only twenty five percent of our total calories. Around every cell there is a cell membrane that contains a little envelope of fat. This is needed for cells to communicate with each other. It is because of this communication ability that the cells are able to react collectively against infection. If this little envelope of fat becomes a big envelope, cell communication becomes muddied. Fat acts like an oil slick on cells, especially on the immune cells, that fight disease and other invaders. It keeps cells from working well. There is a huge difference between fats derived from animal products and fats based on plant seeds and nuts. While beef and pork fat clogs arteries, flax seed oils, sunflower oils, and olive oils all have the opposite effect of lowering cholesterol.

Generally speaking, humans need 25 to 30 grams of fat everyday to build new cells and nerves as well as for other functions, such as healing and restoration. Fats are composed of building blocks called fatty acids. There are three major categories of fatty acids. Meat and dairy products contain saturated fats that clog arteries and are linked with scores of other problems. Vegetable fats are mostly polyunsaturated. They are found in corn, soybeans, sunflower oils, and certain fish oils. This is the healthy kind of fat that plays a role in lowering cholesterol by raising the HDL (high-density lipoprotein) level and reducing inflammation. Monounsaturated fatty acids are found in olive, peanut, canola oils, etc. In excess amounts, they can create problems in the same way as saturated fats. Palm oil and coconut oil are different; they are saturated oils. Though in many tropical areas where these oils are used prolifically, no high rate of heart problems are reported because of their use. It is believed that these oils have some additional elements to neutralize their bad effects. Coconut oil contains lauric acid – the kind found in breast milk along with certain benevolent fatty acids. These fatty acids are quickly metabolized and converted to energy, rather than stored in the body. Through a process called hydrogenation, many vegetable oils are transformed into a solid consistency like butter. Though it might be low in fat, it is capable of raising cholesterol and clogging arteries. These trans fatty acids behave like saturated fats and may raise the

LDL (low-density lipoprotein) cholesterol level. Although most foods contain a combination of all three types of fatty acids, even though one dominates in excess, all may become harmful to the system. Our liver is the storehouse and maker of cholesterol. It is delivered from there to tissues by means of carriers called LDL and transported back to the liver by means of another carrier called HDL. When HDL – the good cholesterol – is lacking, excess cholesterol is not returned to the storehouse, the liver. It is like dumping materials in certain areas with nobody to take care of them. It is this kind of dumping, caused by the lack of carriers, that results in artery clogging.

> ***Fat is our friend and enemy. Fat is vital for our existence. In excess, it contributes to disease and death.***

From all the bad publicity fat has recently drawn from all quarters of the media, one may think that it is our enemy. In fact, fat is vital for our existence. It is necessary for healthy membranes, brain cells, digestion, and the adrenal glands. During infancy and childhood, fat is necessary for normal brain development. Fat is the most concentrated form of energy available to the body. However, after the growing age, it is much less used. Excess fat is stored in the body. Excessive fat intake is a major causative factor in obesity, high blood pressure, coronary heart disease, and colon cancer, and has been linked to a number of other disorders as well.[7] If your cholesterol is abnormal, consider regular exercise, weight control and a diet low in saturated fats. You may need functional foods such as soluble fiber, nuts, green tea, soy, garlic, olive oil, and avocado.

Nutrition

Good nutrition is the foundation of good health. Everyone needs four basic nutrients in a balanced manner in their food intake. They are water, carbohydrates, proteins, and fats. New research and claims have lauded the traditional role of these nutrients. Protein is essential for growth and development. It provides the body energy. Protein is used in the manufacture of hormones, antibodies, enzymes, and tissues. When protein is consumed, the body breaks it down into amino acids, the building blocks of protein. There are essential and non-essential amino acids. Meat, dairy products, poultry, fish, eggs, and milk all complete the protein group that has all of the essential amino acids. But, they are also rich in fat, which has its disadvantages as we have noted. You can look for essential amino acids from other sources that are less harmful. You can have a complete healthy protein diet from the combination of beans with any one of the following: brown rice, corn, nuts, seeds, and wheat. A combination of grains, nuts, seeds, legumes, and a variety of mixed vegetables will make a complete protein diet. All soybean products are complete protein. Yogurt is the only animal-related protein recommended for frequent use. Yogurt contains many friendly bacteria needed for digestion and prevention of some disorders like candidiasis. It also contains vitamins: vitamins A, D, and B-complex.

Carbohydrates are seen more as an enemy to health in recent research and studies. Carbs mainly belong to two groups: simple and complex carbohydrates. Simple carbohydrates are different forms of sugar like fructose, sucrose, lactose, etc. Complex carbohydrates are made of sugars of different types. The molecules are strung to form longer more complex chains. Foods rich in complex carbohydrates include vegetables, whole grain, peas, and beans. Carbohydrates are a source of blood glucose, which is the source of energy for the brain and red blood cells. All carbohydrates are converted into blood glucose. Complex carbs are converted slowly; therefore, they do not raise blood sugar at once or too quickly like simple carbs do. Carbohydrates consumed in a quantity more than present energy needs are converted into body fat. Refined foods that convert easily to energy often produce more than what the body needs at one time. So, they all are converted to fat. And, people often wonder why they become obese when they do not eat much protein or fat. A reduced carbohydrate diet is becoming increasingly popular in developed countries.

Fiber is a very important form of carbohydrate. Fiber is part of plant food that is resistant to digestive enzymes and has some benefits. Fiber retains water, makes softer stools, and prevents constipation and hemorrhoids. A fiber-enriched diet reduces the risk of colon cancer and keeps the digestive tract clean. Fiber binds with certain substances that would normally result in the production of cholesterol. Fiber eliminates these substances from the body. In this way, a high-fiber diet can reduce cholesterol levels, thereby reducing the risk of heart disease. If you eat complex carbohydrates, you will be able to receive the needed fiber.

Two-thirds of the human body consists of water. It helps in transporting nutrients and waste products in and out of cells. Water keeps the body at the right temperature, is used for water-soluble vitamins, and helps in excretory functions. In short, water is the essential nutrient involved in every function of the body. A supply of clean water, eight glasses a day, is a requisite for the healthy functioning of the body. While the body can survive without food for weeks, it cannot survive without water for more than a couple of days. Healthy drinking water has become a luxury item these days. Water may contain many impurities, sometimes naturally and sometimes by preservation methods. Water from certain areas and sources may have arsenic, iron, fluoride, lead, and other heavy metals. Other contaminants like pesticides, herbicides, and industrial chemicals may reach our water in various ways. Chlorine, carbon lime, phosphates, etc. are added by water supply administrations to ensure that there are no bacteria and parasites. These chemicals sometimes go overboard. Though they kill bacteria and parasites, their toxic effect may destroy human cells and lead to many disorders. Residues from pesticides used years ago can reach into the water supply systems and remain for a long period of time.

A clean supply of water for drinking, cooking, and bathing is imperative to maintain good health. Agricultural runoff, manufacturing waste, chlorine, and other chemicals contaminate the water supply system of most cities. When the water supply is contaminated and you drink it, toxic chemicals in the water go right into your bone marrow, fat, and internal organs where they cause distress to the system concerned. Symptoms of pollutants may not manifest themselves immediately. If symptoms had developed, people would have reacted quickly. Problems of poisoning may masquerade as something else and may not be readily traceable to polluted food or water. Whatever may be the source of your water, watch for cloudiness and murkiness as a warning sign. Strange smells and taste indicate chemical contamination. Bacteria can be destroyed if water is boiled for five minutes.

Commercial drinks have made such an impression on the public that water is considered something less valuable to the body than other artificial drinks. Soft drinks have taken the place of drinking water. Pure water serves the body's purpose best. Coffee, tea, soda, or anything that contains caffeine and artificial flavors is no substitute for water. Milk and dairy products as drinks are good only if you are nutritionally starving. Such products are mucous-forming. As people age, many do not have enzymes to break down the milk sugars. Therefore, they experience gas, bloating, diarrhea, etc.

Technology and Food

With the advent of technology, the market is filled with more sophisticated goods and objects. In the dietary field, too much technology has led to the downfall in the quality of foods. Most foods in the market are no longer 'whole' (a term used to describe a food in its most natural and unadulterated form). Processing food with many additives and preservatives has increased the level of many undesirable chemicals in the food. Studies reveal that many additives are linked with heart palpitations, nausea, headaches, and nerve damage. Aspartame, the artificial sweetener used in Nutrasweet, Splenda and Equal, can cause headaches, migraines, rashes, insomnia, and loss of motor control, etc., according to the Food and Drug Administration in the United States. The effects of many substitutes and additives have not been fully researched or documented. When a food is processed or refined, it loses its nutritional punch. In the end, food will be left with less vitamins, minerals, and fiber, and instead remain with more fat, sugar, and salt, which leads to more troubles over the course of time.

Untreated fresh meat, vegetables, and fruits rarely fill most modern markets. Fruits and vegetables are routinely grown with artificial fertilizers, sprayed with pesticides, and treated with hormones. Chemicals are used to control the time of ripening and mechanical harvesting. They are dyed and sprayed with chemicals to prevent ripening during the period they are transported and sit on the supermarket shelves. A good number of fruits are coated with waxes to give a glossy appearance. Most of the breads that come to market do not have nutritional value. Rice, wheat, and other whole grains provide a rich source of nutrients, complex carbohydrates, proteins, and fiber, as well as an excellent balance of vitamins and minerals. Since food has become an industry, bakers make products that can be packed, shipped, and kept for a longer period of time. This necessitates processing and adding preservatives. Sometimes, the products are enriched by a synthetic version of vitamins, which in no way is equal to the original vitamins and nutrients that are lost in the processing.

Commercially grown animals and fowl are fed with synthetic vitamins, minerals, and antibiotics. Drugs used in their foods reduce their physical activity to a minimum, thus saving on feed. Plant crops are also manipulated in various ways. Fruits and vegetables are grown in nutrient-depleted soil with lavish artificial fertilizers and treated with poisonous chemicals, most of which are carcinogenic. The chemicals absorbed by the plants can never be washed away completely, as they have already gone into the cellular structure of the stems and leaves. No amount of cooking and rinsing can destroy these chemicals, and they are passed along to us as we eat these foods. It is a wonder that many of us still keep our health!

These days, you are not able to readily get simple natural salt. Sea salt contains a spectrum of minerals. But, unfortunately, it is rarely available in an unrefined form. In the unrefined form, it is gray, lumpy, and draws moisture easily (gray salt is also very costly). So, we make salt beautiful to our eyes, easy to handle, and presentable at our dining tables. Extracted oils and fats are deficient in the same manner. You do not get complementary vitamins as a benefit from the product. They become fuels lifted out of their normal context. Oils, when cooked, produce free radicals that damage cells, finally leading to malignancies. Eating whole foods and storing some of their excess as fat is a very different process than taking extracted fat from whole foods and discarding the remainder of the plant or animal. So far, there is no evidence that tells us that humans need more fats and oils than what one gets from eating natural and/or organic foods.

Dietary Mindfulness

Food is not a mere source of energy; it is a healing agent, too. The reason for so many sicknesses can be traced to the wrong food and nutritional imbalance of the food along with the toxic elements contained in it. Minutes after you eat, molecules of food are in every cell of your body. There they produce changes in every level of your body from the pH level in your blood to the membrane changes in your muscles and nerves. To maintain health, you must eat with mindfulness by sharpening your sense of what is right for you. It is necessary to pay close attention to your body and its cues. Eat mindfully, relishing it, and listening to the subtle messages each food gives. In eating, one must evaluate the food in terms of one's constitution and energy needs. Eat only those things you really need. Because the clock indicates it is time for food, or the food being served could be wasted, these are not good reasons to eat when you are really not in need of food. You may have to eat whatever is placed before you when you are starving and in need of energy for daily functions. But, when you are in a situation to make a choice, choose whole foods with less salt, sugar, and fat, tailoring your intake to suit your constitution and needs. Many are in the habit of consuming nutritionally and calorically imbalanced food.

There is no ideal foodstuff fit for all. Your constitutionality and requirements of the moment are the determining factors.

What you eat can affect your consciousness. The Eastern dietary system had explored this in depth centuries ago.[8] There are contractive foods and expansive foods. Contractive foods make your internal systems tighter and make you more compressed physically and mentally. Expansive foods do just the opposite. Salt is contractive and sugar is expansive. There are hyperactive foods that whip up rapid thought, restlessness, and speedy actions, such as coffee, hot spicy foods, red meat, etc. According to Vedic traditions there are rajasic, tamasic, and sattvic foods. Rajasic food is the food of the king – food fit for a king – for aggression, conquest, and activity. Natural fresh meat is rajasic, but when it is processed and kept long, it develops a quality that is dark and heavy. It is then tamasic. Most of the fast foods in the market are tamasic. Food that is flavored and kept a long time on the shelves loses its energetic quality to nourish you on the spiritual-subtle energetic level. Today, people consume more quantity of foods than in earlier decades, but the energetic quality of the food is poor. Eating tamasic foods clouds consciousness and affects the resonance of subtle energies. Conversely, sattvic foods facilitate healing and give clarity to thoughts and the mental state. This will be discussed further later in this chapter.

According to the Ayurvedic traditions, everything on this planet is composed of five elements: Earth, Water, Fire, Air and Ether. Every form of life contains these elements in varying proportions. The Earth element predominates, giving structure to the cell. The Water element predominates in the cytoplasm. The metabolic process regulating the cell is governed mainly by the Fire element. The Air element predominates in the gases of the cell. The space occupied by the cell represents Ether. One might think of the assimilation of food as a process of a sifting through, gleaning the more subtle elements to nourish and sustain the higher vibrations of your consciousness; using some portions of the grosser elements to bolster physical existence; and finally discarding the excess of these grosser elements as feces and urine.[9]

Consciousness is the product of subtle energy patterns. What you eat can have a potent impact on how your brain functions. The brain uses nutrients, such as vitamin B12, thiamin, niacin, choline and folic acid to enhance brain function. The brain needs minerals like copper, iron, and zinc that are thought to influence the function of nerve endings. In addition, the brain uses electrolytes, such as sodium, potassium, calcium, and magnesium to transmit electrical signals between cells.

Fresh, live food possesses most elements needed for the brain. It has a vibrancy and resonance that can support consciousness and its energy patterns. Sattvic foods are the fresh fruits and vegetables, rice, beans, nuts and seeds, and milk from healthy animals. Whether you are led to a sattvic state of consciousness depends on if you select foods based on your needs and physical constitution. Even the most ideal foodstuffs must be put through the filter of your constitutionality and requirement of the moment. If that is done, there occurs a congruence or resonance between your body and the food ingested, and thereby, the food assumes a corrective quality or medicinal power.

Not all Foods are Food

Nature has provided ample foods to nurture and sustain human health. Love the natural and what nature provides. Exclude, if possible, all dairy products and processed foods. Avoid refined carbohydrates, simple sugars, flavor enhancers, color enhancers, artificial preservatives, foods treated with pesticides, and artificial sweeteners. Minimize the use of coffee and tea. They may be replaced with pure water or green teas. Avoid altogether carbonated soft drinks. At a glance, these suggestions all may sound too restrictive. Your feeling is such mainly because of the narrow range of food items to which you are accustomed. A wide variety of food items are there in nature from which you can select. Taste is something you develop through the years. If you are convinced about the advantage of a wide variety of foods and motivate yourself, you will slowly develop taste buds accordingly. Our food style is culturally and commercially conditioned. People from different cultures manifest different tastes for food. I have heard people say: 'I just want to eat normal food.' The commercialization of food created false flavors and appearances that resulted in a greater appeal for them rather than natural foods.

What we need to maintain good health is the simple food that nature provides. They include a wide selection of whole grains, nuts, seeds, fruits, legumes, fresh herbs, etc. Nature nurtures and heals people who are in love with nature's gifts. A change in diet is the first step one can take to effect health by natural means. Change in diet requires courage and determination. Stepping out of an unhealthy dietary pattern is a radical step towards health building. Studies have consistently revealed that reducing the level of calories consumed can significantly increase the span of health. Phytochemicals found in edible plants have been understood to have potential benefits in the prevention and treatment of disease. Phytochemicals are found in many foods, especially fruits and vegetables.

Leaving nature's gifts, people seek vitamin pills. The number of vitamin bottles on the shelves of health stores and pharmacies has quadrupled. The body is not designed to accept substitutes readily. Crops produced by highly mechanized means repeatedly in the same soil with artificial fertilizers do not possess the many required nutrients and minerals. Then, whatever nutritional value remains is reduced further by the processing and other commercial methods used in packaging and shipping. Since the nutrients have disappeared from food, another food industry rose to fill the vacuum – the vitamin industry. There is a joke about vitamin consumers: 'if you take vitamin pills, you will get more costly urine.' The body does not absorb most synthetic vitamins. They are supplements, not substitutes. Instead, the natural whole food bears some complex and immediate relation to the digestive tract and human physiology. Therefore, the natural vitamins from nature's supply are the best way to get all the vitamins you need. In the Ayurvedic tradition, there is a remarkable saying: 'If you have a good diet, of what use is a doctor; if you don't have a good diet, what use is a doctor?'

Sinful Cravings

Sugar, salt, and fat have an appealing taste for most of humanity. That which appeals to our taste and desires can be easily abused by going overboard in its use. Sugar is the center of the energy economy. Natural whole foods are packaged with nutrients to burn the sugar effectively. Natural foods come with an appropriate complement of vitamins and minerals. Taking sugar alone or extracting sugar alone from wholesome food is equal to cheating nature. You are thwarting nature's wisdom and design for its pleasurable aspects. Too much sugar in the blood stresses the pancreas because it has to produce more insulin to absorb the sugar. Simple carbohydrates or sugar blast the blood stream with glucose. Repeated episodes can exhaust the insulin-secreting cells and lead to difficulty in regulating blood sugars. The result is hypoglycemia or diabetes. Sugar can produce dramatic behavioral changes. The ability to remain calm and the power to concentrate are affected by sugar consumption. Kids become hyperactive and develop trouble in learning. Excess sugar in the intestinal tract attracts an overgrowth of yeast. The yeast ferments the sugar, producing gas and bloating.

In the early centuries, sugar was a luxury and costly, so consumption was very minimal. A good number of commercial food products give extra flavor with sugar coating. Cakes and sweets have become part of everyday life. Often, cakes are coated liberally in frosting with sugar. Colored sugar water – soft drinks – has become the fashion.

Most people take into their body more than the needed amount of salt. 'I don't have any blood pressure problem, so I am OK with salt' is not a tenable argument. There are certain biochemical reasons to limit the amount of salt to the minimum. You need to balance the sodium-potassium level in the body. Potassium is the positively charged ion in the cell. Sodium is its extra-cellular counterpart. When sodium collects, it holds excess water in the tissues. It begins to invade the cell and replaces the potassium. This will undermine conduction of the nerve impulses. Excess salts may create malignancies, too. We have already discussed how fats and oils extracted from their natural context lack nutrients to burn them properly. Most creams, sauces, and gravies contain large amounts of fats and oils. The food you ingest can make or break you sooner or later. Dietary mindfulness can produce a miraculous amount of prevention, protection, and healing in our bodies.

Vegetarianism

Scientific studies reveal the adequacy and superiority of organic vegetarianism. It is not difficult to see that fruits, vegetables, and whole grains have a greater power to build and restore our body. Most cancers are diet related. Organic fruits and vegetables can get rid of cancerous cells and can rejuvenate the body. The higher content of fiber in a vegetarian diet is the basis for many of its advantages. Fiber has the ability to collect and pull toxic substances out of the body. Vegetarianism is desirable economically and ecologically. The cost of meat is relatively high in most places of the economy. There are no proportionate benefits, but, on the other hand, considerable disadvantages. The intake of toxic chemicals dramatically drops in organic vegetarianism. Heart attack is seven times greater with meat eaters. Cancer, arthritis, and osteoporosis are much less likely to occur in those who do not eat meat. Meat is believed to promote aggression and competition. So, it may give you an edge in the competitive worlds of sports, business, etc.

It has been established that to a great extent the right diet can protect you against certain diseases such as cancer, heart disease, hypertension, high blood pressure, arthritis, diabetes, and problems related with obesity. I am not advocating that if you become a vegetarian, good health is guaranteed. However, it definitely pays off. Fruits, vegetables, legumes, and whole grains are nutrient-dense. This means they are extremely low in fat while being high in fiber and have key nutrients that can help protect you against illness and, likewise, may even treat illness. Barbara Clein wrote in *The Journal of Food Medicine,* "While you could get the nutrients you need from taking vitamin supplements, the advantage to getting them in the fruits and vegetables is that you get other micronutrients that you can't get in a pill." Trace minerals and other compounds are believed to play a key role in protecting one against certain diseases, and possibly even healing them. Among these are phytochemicals, which are the natural chemicals formed in all plants. They protect the plants against too much sunlight, disease, and being eaten by other animals. The phytochemicals that help plants might help humans, too, against disease and build immunity. Citrus fruits contain bioflavanoids that prevent cancer-causing hormones from latching on to cells. Green pepper and pineapple have substances that stop cancer cells from forming. Different phytochemicals in the tomato can play an important role in stopping tumors before they form. It is the immune system that fights colds and infection. If you eat right, your immunity stays strong irrespective of your age.

Exercise

One low-tech way to keep healthy and live longer is to exercise. You may be eating well nutritionally and avoiding caffeine, alcohol, and smoking. Still, if you do not exercise, you may not achieve optimum health. There was a time when people thought vigorous exercise was needed to maintain health. Exercises that involve steady rhythmic motions of major muscles that burn oxygen can be considered as aerobic exercises. Aerobic exercises increase the heart rate. This, in turn, increases the blood circulation that brings more oxygen to muscles. Swimming, bicycle riding, jogging, and power walking are aerobic exercises that can improve the body's capacity to use fuel and oxygen. Twenty minutes a day can keep the heart healthy and lower blood pressure. Anaerobic exercise, light weight-lifting, is the isolated movement of muscles. It increases muscle size and strength but does not necessarily oxygenate the blood. Walking is convenient and gentle exercise for people of all ages and all levels. It helps boost metabolism as the heart rate increases the circulation of blood, oxygen, and nutrients to all parts of the body tissues. As the muscles contract and relax, you utilize minerals such as magnesium and potassium. Running has an advantage of flushing toxins from the system. It can also reduce stress that is triggering so many of the illnesses today.

Exercise is a first-class ticket to good health. Doctors do not use exercise as a treatment modality, but it is the first line of defense. Inactivity is hazardous to one's health. Some of the major benefits of exercise are worth mentioning in order to have a keen awareness of its significance, namely:

- Reduces heart problems
- Trims unwanted pounds
- Maintains weight loss
- Lowers blood pressure
- Relieves lower back pain
- Eases arthritis, menstrual discomfort
- Eases depression, boosts self-esteem
- Lessens incidents of colds and flu
- Increases energy levels
- Reduces stress
- Results in fewer sleep problems
- Improves digestion and relieves constipation
- Strengthens bones and burns extra calories

Fitness is a life-long commitment. The physical benefits of being fit and staying fit are numerous. By honoring your commitment and following it, you increase your self-worth and provide for a better self-image. Exercise is not merely physical. It also has spiritual and mental benefits. When you exercise with love and commitment, it can help you to connect with your deepest self.

Life is constituted of different movements from within to without. When you move physically, life flows. When you move, energy flows in all directions. The energy dynamism makes you dynamic. Kierkegaard remarked, "Depression is what occurs when the spirit wants to move you and you resist." When there is no movement, bound-up energy begins to stress your muscles and nerves. Because of the mind-body interaction, the body's stress makes the mind lethargic. Decades earlier, the genius of Gandhi realized the energetic nature of the body and its relation to body movements. He said, "Exercise is as much of a vital necessity for man as air, water, and food. The mind is weakened by want of exercise as is the body."[10]

Detoxification

Toxicity is a major health concern. Health is increasingly being threatened by the use of powerful chemicals, air and water pollution, and radiation. There are now more than 100,000 synthetic chemicals available in worldwide markets today, and each year the quantity is swelling. What their impact is on health is not yet fully known. Dangerous pesticides are still in common use in many countries. Although the human system is very resilient and can tolerate a good deal of environmental toxins, it has its limits.

As the use of drugs increases, more chemicals are ingested into our body. Sugar, refined foods, stimulants, and sedatives all create toxic waste in the body. High salt and high protein diets leave strong concentrated residues that stress kidneys. Internally, the body produces toxins through everyday metabolism. However, a mineral-depleted soil does not provide the needed trace minerals for a healthy metabolism. This also has raised the toxic level in the body. Biochemical and cellular activities generate substances that need to be eliminated. Proper elimination of toxins is critical. If not eliminated, they will stress the immune system and the healthy function of the body. Toxicity occurs when we ingest more toxins than we can utilize and eliminate. Toxins may produce a rapid onset of symptoms or they may cause slow, long-term effects. The cleansing process will encourage the immune system. The general detoxification systems of humans are:

- Gastrointestinal – liver, gallbladder, colon and the whole GI tract
- Urinary – kidneys, bladder and urethra
- Respiratory – lungs, bronchial tubes, throat, sinuses and nose
- Lymphatic – lymph channels and lymph nodes
- Skin and dermal – sweat and sebaceous glands and tears

Our body handles toxins either by neutralizing, transforming, or eliminating them. Antioxidants such as vitamin C, beta-carotene, selenium, and vitamin E all enjoy the power to neutralize free-radical molecules. The liver is constantly at work transforming toxic substances into harmless ones. The liver also sends waste through the bile into the intestines where it is eliminated. When you sweat by heat or exercise, the body has an outlet to disperse some waste through the sweat glands.

Toxicity symptoms are many. They include headache, fatigue, congestion, swollen joints, obesity, allergy, and sensitivity to all environmental changes. To maintain good health, the five elimination systems in our body should function optimally. Though each individual system is important, the intestinal health system is central to the overall health of the body. A diet rich in fiber is essential for the smooth functioning of the intestines. Fiber helps prevent the absorption of cholesterol and fat from the intestinal tract. By avoiding fats, using organic foods, minimizing contact with plastic-packaged foods, and avoiding pesticides in the home environment and garden, you can fortify your body's cleansing system.

Lifestyle Problems

Our cleansing systems are handicapped by our lifestyle. Increasingly, many cultures tend to emphasize external cleanliness. Every institution has standard sanitary procedures and environments that they like to keep or enforce. Hardly any culture emphasizes internal cleanliness, being considered as something private. Partly by ignorance and partly by laziness, most people do not have internal cleanliness. One reason for a messy, unclean situation in our bodies is our tendency to overeat and undereliminate. Unwanted, unused things make clutter to the whole system. They are collected in the less important areas of the body, often in the extremities. It is this kind of clutter that makes joints stiff and painful. If we are dealing with moderate levels of waste and pollutants, the basic routes of excretion – colon, kidney, skin, lungs – can comfortably handle all necessary elimination. Unfortunately, modern life has greatly burdened these elimination channels.

The prevalence of food that is highly processed and preserved with additives has contributed to a sluggish elimination process. Besides, the colon is poorly equipped because of the heavy use of antibiotics and sugar. Constipation is a common complaint for many. A low-fiber diet and the sub-optimal intake of water, as well as a lack of exercise due to the sedentary nature of work, have weakened bowel movements in many people. Social gatherings and parties are on the rise. At these events, individuals proportionately ingest more alcohol, coffee, sugar-laden desserts, and high-fat protein products. Thus far, sufficient thought has not been given to serving healthy food at various social gatherings and dinners. Sometimes mental and emotional factors are also involved in constipation. Constipation and obesity reveal the tendency to hold on to old relationships, possessions, thoughts or memories.

Sometimes cleansing of the bowel can catalyze the release of mental, emotional and physical remains stored over the years. Colon cleansing is one of the most important steps in detoxification.

Detox diets, supplements, laxatives, enemas, fasting, and juice cleansing are some methods used to clean the GI tract. Perspiration is a means employed by the body to clear toxins from the body. The body can throw out smelly, foul things through our skin. Sadly, we have found ways to block this process. Modern life cleverly caps the sweat glands by deodorants. They constrict the pores. To make up for the capped sweat glands, the body's recourse is the mucous membranes. Mucus is produced in the related tissues to moisten and protect the organs. It is mainly seen around the mouth, nose, eyes, vagina, and rectum. When all channels are blocked, mucous membranes provide an outlet. Excessive mucus in concerned organs is sometimes an alternate outlet. The skin needs vigorous exercise if it is to work at its optimum. Naturopathy encourages the brushing of the skin with a natural bristle brush. It helps to open pores and stimulate the breakdown and removal of materials deposited in the connective tissue spaces. You can increase elimination through the lungs by breathing more fully and by strengthening the diaphragm.

When the cumulative load of environmental toxins and metabolic waste exceeds the body's capacity to throw off toxins, the first place they go is in the space between the cells. Some body mechanism envelops it there in the extra-cellular space without disrupting normal cellular life. When this extra-cellular space runs out, one may experience stiffness caused by the deposits and pain throughout the body. It is rheumatism. Fibromyalgia is just another form of rheumatic disorder characterized by chronic achy muscular pain. New and fashionable names of diseases do not change the basic nature of illness. Extra-cellular space is the first stop-off for all sorts of metabolic dross including protein substances. Fat-soluble toxic materials end up in fatty tissue, cholesterol in the arterial walls, and stones in the gallbladder. Minerals are usually deposited in the joint spaces or become kidney or bladder stones. Much of what we consider as aging has less to do with age than with the progressive accumulation of toxic materials.

The liver is the center of metabolic activities for the body. It contains many enzymes responsible for metabolism. It is responsible for the detox process. The liver converts and mobilizes toxins into forms that can be easily discharged. Everything that comes from the intestinal surface first goes to the liver. It is a stopover point where toxins are pulled out, nutrients are sorted, and essentials are stored for future use. It is the responsibility of the liver to filter out and package all chemical pollutants that are ingested through water, air, food, etc. If the liver is overburdened, toxins are accumulated, which invite microbial growth and disease. The liver needs nutrients to discharge its duties.

Maintenance of Cleansing Organs

- Colon – exercise; high-fiber diet; water
- Urinary tract – water; diet low in fat, salt, and protein
- Skin – water; aerobics
- Lungs – complete breath; fresh air

Fasting for Cleansing

Nourishing and cleansing are the two sides of the health coin. If you inhale, you have to exhale. When you nourish, you make use of certain mechanisms in your body. Constant work will make the body's mechanism messy, stressed, and worn out. Therefore, if you do not give sufficient attention to cleansing and needed rest, those organs needed for your health will fail. Fasting is believed to be the single greatest natural healing therapy. Animals with an illness do not eat anything, and even if they eat, they eat very sparingly until they are restored. Fasting is a useful personal tool that can touch the inner core of the person and, as such, it has been valued in all spiritual traditions. It is a powerful tool to enliven the spirit and to let new energies flow into the body. Most people have an instinctive fear of fasting. They fear they might collapse, and it will bring up more problems. A planned fasting revitalizes the body and will be a solution for many medical and life problems. When congestion and clutter in the body are cleared, the mind draws more clarity. The body is attuned to the spirit and its purpose and, thereby, greater intuition and creativity will surface. This is why Gandhi often resorted to fasting especially when he was challenged by numerous problems. The Bible said it more clearly: "One does not live by bread alone, but by every word that comes forth from the mouth of God." (Matthew 4:4) One will be able to receive God's communication doubly when bodies are attuned to the spirit by fasting.

When nourishing is stopped, then the flurry of cleansing starts up. Since cleansing is a task, it needs energy; the liver needs to be boosted with vitamins and minerals to do the work. Juice fasting is, therefore, most beneficial; it can eliminate much of the trauma of fasting as well as allow nutrients to do the cleansing work. Fasting becomes starvation if you feel drained, depleted and exhausted. Fasting correctly brings rejuvenation and cellular repair. Freshly squeezed and extracted vegetable juices and fruits contain a wealth of vitamins and minerals. Fresh juice has a cleansing effect. Four glasses of light juice a day will keep you going and help do the cleansing work. Drinking more than 500 calories a day is not good when you are juice fasting. Fasting two or more days will mobilize the toxins and fat deposits. As they enter the bloodstream, taking extra water will help to flush them out. Vitamin C, pantothenic acid, several amino acids, and glutathione are found to help step-up the cleansing process. Fasting is a slow, gradual, and more comprehensive cleansing, unlike enemas and colonics, whose effect is short and immediate. It is better to start fasting slowly, preferably by taking raw vegetables and fruits on the first day.

Though cleansing is crucial to health, orthodox medicine widely ignores it. Scientific medicine discarded it as unscientific though all cultures found wisdom in cleansing. Flooding the toxic-laden body with antibiotics and other medicine is like spraying in a dirty kitchen to get rid of bugs and vermin. To break the habit of eating three meals and two snacks is a challenge for many. Initially, one may feel withdrawal symptoms when the stomach is empty. This will pass after the initial day. Nutritionally, fasting helps us appreciate the more subtle aspects of our diet, as less food and simple flavors will become more satisfying.[11] After fasting, you will definitely experience greater energy and freshness. Results and experience may vary among people based on their personalities; nevertheless, fasting is a multi-dimensional experience worth trying. Fasting combined with spiritual practices can bring even greater benefits.

What has been said so far boils down to one vital truth. Food is medicinal. Food that creates a free-flow of bodily functions builds health and wards off disease. When bodily functions are congested by toxic foods with depleted nutrients and excessive calories, our system gets stressed. When body systems are stressed internally, they will have a difficult time handling stress externally. Achieving health over disease requires removing the above-discussed causative factors.

7

The Health Approach of Homeopathy

I know there are people who are skeptical and totally opposed to homeopathy. And, there are those who have almost a mystical belief in its curative powers. There also are reasonable people who view it as another therapeutic model that can have some beneficial results. I, myself, had no faith in this medicine. From my childhood to my late thirties, I suffered from frequent colds, otitis media, and sinus infections. Having been treated with conventional medicine by various specialists in the field for many long years, I finally underwent surgery for my ear problem and another surgery for my sinus. Both surgeries having proved to be of no avail, I stopped all treatments. And then, I got interested in complementary medicines and took a course in homeopathy. At the end of the course, I tried the remedies on myself. I treated myself with homeopathic medicine, mercury 6c, for a couple of weeks. To my surprise, I found immediate relief and a lasting cure from my problems. Homeopathic treatments are too good to be true!

In light of the discoveries of modern physics, its theories are much more intelligible and meaningful.

Allopathy vs. Homeopathy

Many medical scientists even today continue to insist that homeopathy has no scientific foundation and, therefore, has no power to bring curative results. Hundreds of studies and researches have proven the efficacy of homeopathy in bringing total cure to the patients where allopathy (conventional medicine) has failed. But, by maintaining that only material things can make an impact on the human body, medical science eliminates a whole spectrum of healing methods that offers healing and hope to the needy.

The germ theory, which states that there is a malevolent microbe behind every disease and it can be vanquished by antibiotics, intoxicated medical science in the beginning of the nineteenth century. Miraculous results were brought into the arena of infectious diseases. The euphoria did not prevail long. The latter part of the twentieth century witnessed the advent of many chronic illnesses that could not be explained by the germ theory. There are microbes present everywhere; no place is devoid of them. However, they are not active everywhere in spite of their pervasive presence. A disordered or disorganized tissue becomes the breeding ground for vigorous action of infectious agents. Some kind of subtle energy derangement in the system brings them on.

Most disease involves disorder on multiple levels; the proliferation of a bacteria, fungus, or virus is merely one physical manifestation of a multilevel, complex disturbance. If this is true, then virtually every disease will be found to have a typical psychological picture, a distinctive energetic derangement, a well-defined metabolic or biochemical expression, and a characteristic microbe that tends to grow.[1] Without taking into consideration this multidimensionality of the human being, no healing will be complete.

To have a total healing, it is not enough to know what microbes are present. It is not enough to know what is the present status of a tissue or organ. One must explore what mental and spiritual stress contributed to the energy derangement and inviting of the microbes. Scientific medicine is not concerned with what went before. They see only the end result that is the symptom. Attacking the symptom and overcoming it is the medical model of allopathy. Though it claims itself scientific, this method is not truly scientific.

I am convinced that every medical discipline deserves attention and needs to be explored in an unbiased manner. One may not find all wisdom in a single medical discipline. Ayurveda, acupuncture, and chiropractic care all have their own separate advantages. What works for one, may not work in the same fashion to effect healing in another. We are individuals with our own individual properties and characteristics. Our sickness also has this individual characteristic. No therapy works all the time for all individuals. Homeopathy is a very individual-oriented therapeutic, which when properly applied, can bring healing to many kinds of diseases. Conventional medicine is best used in certain situations and especially in acute cases or emergency conditions. For example, using an inhaler during an asthma attack can save a life, but it cannot take the problem away. You can ward off infection by the use of antibiotics. But, if you are suffering from frequent infections, you must look elsewhere in order to boost your immune system.

The scientific aura of modern medicine leads many to disregard all other disciplines as outdated or irrelevant. Scientific medicine has not been as scientific as we may think. Even in conventional medicine, most treatments and drug therapies are out of date and replaced within a few years. We have noted earlier some of the follies and foibles of these medicines. Being rightly informed about other medical traditions may help to approach them with the right attitudes and beliefs so that the healing benefits may be largely increased. This fact has been clinically proven effective in chronic cases without any side effects. A quick survey of the principles and laws involved in the homeopathic system helps one know where to look to find the needed help. The willingness to consider other therapies is beginning to spread, even in the scientific West.

Every medical discipline has its own understanding of what causes sickness, and what cures it. Medical science treats the disease, disregarding the person behind it, because it is materialistic in nature. Homeopathy expresses a different approach. It has a distinctive understanding of health and healing that recognizes the integrity of the whole person. Homeopathy developed a medical approach that works dynamically, integrating different elements. It does not disregard the body as many spiritualists do. Neither does it disregard the spirit as many materialists do. Homeopathy respects the hierarchy and role of every element that constitutes the human being to achieve wholeness. In a complex organism like man, health is the result of a dynamic equilibrium of different elements, giving the appearance of rest while based in constant change. The achievement of balance adds an extra quality to the organism that we refer to as *'wholeness'*.

Founder's Vision

In the eighteenth and nineteenth centuries, scientific medicine made tremendous leaps in discovery, but the healing disciplines continued on a primitive level. This period was known as the 'age of heroic medicine' because of the reckless vigor of its methods. There were no laws or principles formulated to govern therapeutics. It was during this time that Samuel Hahnemann, a German doctor, formulated, for the first time in the history of medicine, the complete laws and principles governing health and disease and proved them in actual clinical trials. He found that medicines were too invasive and accomplished little. He felt the need for a different type of healing method and medical philosophy. Being a deeply religious man, Hahnemann believed that healing comes from God and nature and needed only to be gently encouraged by the physician.[2] He expounded a holistic approach to health and healing in his book *Organon.*

He believed it was unethical to give drugs that have not been self-tested. In his genuineness and spirit, he set out to prove the common remedies of his day on himself, following the careful rules he had devised. His spiritual beliefs led him to consider that spiritual reality may be more important than physical reality. Applying this attitude to therapeutics, he came to regard the spiritual essence of the drug more important than its physical substance.

In good health, he took a dose of the bark of the cinchona and found it made him feverish. This experience was later reinforced by many experiments, with many substances, and gave him the first part of the theory that he called the Law of Similars. What it means is that a substance, which produces a certain set of symptoms in a healthy person, has the power to cure the sick person manifesting those same symptoms. He coined the term 'homeopathy' to refer to his new method of treatment. His philosophy, combined with the results of his experiments, brought him to the *law of infinitesimal.* This means that a smaller dose of the remedy, the more diluted and successed, (the vigorous shaking method according to the rules of homeopathy), the more effective it will be at stimulating the body's vital forces to react against diseases. Recognition of an internal spiritual principle is nothing new. It has almost been universal in all cultures. Homeopathy has brought this internal spiritual principle into the healing realm, exploring it in depth and breadth. Different philosophies have named this spiritual principle differently as spirit, energy, Vital Force, etc.

Homeopathy is based on the belief that a human being does not get sick in part. Rather, it is the whole of an individual – body, mind, and spirit – that becomes sick. The symptoms expressed by the mind and body are simply signs that there is an imbalance in the force that binds the three together.

The Vital Force Theory

The philosophy of vitalism postulates that an intelligent power within governs the myriads of processes that maintain the being in existence as it passes through different environments and phases. To an objective observer, it is obvious that some force animates the body, because the human organism is much more than the sum of its parts. Some animating principle enters the body at the inception of life, guides all the functions of life, and leaves it at the time of death. At death, an organism is structurally intact, but something that coordinated and animated the various actions is lacking.

According to the theory of vitalism, the body is composed of a hierarchy of parts – cells, tissues, and organs. These parts, or systems, are fully interdependent in both ascending and descending order, and their relationship to one another is controlled by a steering entity – the Vital Force. Under normal conditions, the Vital Force is thought to be responsible for the orderly and harmonious functions of the body and for coordinating the body's defense against disease. It dominates the life process within the biological environment and controls the quality of the body's vibration. This controlling force can become disturbed by many factors such as stress, poor diet, allergies, drugs, polluted environment, etc. The disturbance of the Vital Force experience is expressed in the form of symptoms in the body that we call 'sickness'. The Vital Force is increasingly reacting to its environment to ward off danger and repair damage. So, what is called 'sickness' is actually the Vital Force's attempt to restore order and health. Illnesses are the Vital Force's reaction to disturbing factors that affect its vibratory rhythm.

The Vital Force operates on three different vibratory levels: mental, emotional, and physical. The three planes may be depicted as a set of concentric circles with the mental plane, the most fundamental, being represented by the innermost circle. Homeopathic remedies are intended to restore the vibratory level of the Vital Force that is disturbed by some morbific stimulus. If a patient consults a homeopath for asthma, and only the physical symptoms, such as shortness of breath, are taken into account in the prescription, while ignoring the emotional and mental symptoms, the prescription is likely to act only locally (on the physical vibratory level). Such a procedure will not give a total cure. To be effective, any medicine should be chosen according to the patient's total symptoms. It is postulated that the resonance of a homeopathic remedy affects the resonance of the Vital Force.[3] The chemistry and structure of the physical body are influenced by the substances and energies from the subtle level.

In light of modern physics and the quantum theory, the Vital Force can be likened to a field similar or analogous to the electromagnetic field.[4] The electromagnetic field is the interrelationship of particles affecting each other through change and movement. These relationships are definable in terms of vibrations. The vibration of a complex organism is highly complex in frequency, regularity, and amplitude. This is why the Vital Force level of the human organism is considered the dynamic plane, affecting all levels of being at once with varying degrees of harmony and strength.[5] A change in the vibration of the Vital Force occurs when the organism is exposed to viruses, bacteria, environmental pressures, harsh drugs, etc. Antibiotics and suppressive medicines alter the vibrational rhythm in the Vital Force. The new resonant frequency makes the patient vulnerable to new disease. The principle of resonance renders the organism susceptible to the influence basically on only one level at any given time. Each level represents susceptibility to a particular range of diseases. A psychotic person is less likely to acquire an acute illness. This is because the resonant frequency of the Vital Force is at a deeper level – mental – and the Vital Force simply does not have the force to react on a peripheral level. Generally, patients with a chronic ailment are immune to other serious illnesses. Once the resonant frequency has changed, susceptibility of the organism to disease has also changed.

In medical treatments, you feel recovery from particular symptoms, but you do not feel an internal sense of well-being. You may have developed an immunity from a particular disturbance, but you are susceptible to more morbific diseases by having the resonance changed. If the Vital Force and its vibrations are too weak, it cannot bring out any symptoms externally, and the person will be sick internally. We noted earlier that symptoms are messengers. They are the body's attempt to heal. A curative action occurs because the treatment resonates with the level of susceptibility of the organ at that moment. Any therapeutic agent that can act on the dynamic plane of the Vital Force – its electromagnetic field – can bring about a cure. Since the Vital Force and its electromagnetic field are a subtle energy and a subtle field, an element of such a nature can only influence it and lead to a cure. The genius of homeopathy has realized this truth in its curative efforts.

Materialistic science cannot recognize homeopathy, for it is based on subtle energies and vibrations science cannot measure.

The vibratory level of crude medicine is foreign to the Vital Force, and it can derange the mechanism for all time to come. Those of you who have tested homeopathy already know that it contains no crude substances or chemicals. Homeopathy's potentized medicine contains a subtle energy to influence the Vital Force. The method of making the medicine is such that it finally has no chemical particle or atom of the original substance but only its energy. Materialistic science and medicine have difficulty in accepting this fact. According to these disciplines, that which you cannot measure does not enjoy any value or truth. Homeopathic medicines that do not contain any atom of the original substance by which each one is named have been proven effective in scores of cases. A spiritually-evolved person, by his laying of hands, can effect a cure because he radiates a subtle energy to influence the resonance of the Vital Force. The symptoms and signs that the Vital Force give out are clues to effect healing. It is a way of drawing attention to the malady.

In allopathy, it is the material aspect of the medicine that counts. Homeopathy uses natural substances that contain no drug materials because it believes that it works in the dynamic spiritual plane. The true nature of man is spiritual; spirit is the essence, and it is prior to the body and enlivens the body. The cause of maladies cannot be material because the least foreign material substance, however mild it may be, is suddenly repelled like a poison by the Vital Force.

In many instances, doctors cannot come up with any diagnosis and are confused about the nature of the disease. There is nothing measurable and visible to be accounted for. The patient still complains that he is sick. As long as no tissue changes, allopathy sees no problem in the patient. Homeopathy understands it differently. It takes into account what a person feels, thinks, tastes, craves, experiences, etc., because this shows the nature of the internal realm. It is the internal principle that changes prior to the body. Homeopaths recognize that the muscles, nerves, ligaments, and other parts of one's physical frame are a picture that manifests to the intelligent physician the internal man.[6] The recognition of this internal principle is critical to the homeopathic philosophy and application. Hahnemann, the founder of homeopathy, remarks, "When a person falls ill, it is only the spiritual automatic Vital Force everywhere present in the organs that is primarily deranged by the dynamic influence upon it of a morbific agent inimical to life."[7]

Healing Principles

From what has been discussed so far, it is obvious that it is the interior of man that is disordered in sickness and not primarily tissues. When the disorder in the internal realm is translated to the external – we have bodily symptoms. So, the bodily symptoms are at the end of a spectrum. A topsy-turvy understanding and treatment cannot bring healing in a complex organism, such as a human being. Since the interior economy was deranged first, it should be mended first. Briefly, in considering treatment, the focus must be on the internal principle first and the external principle last. The principle of cure in homeopathy is based on this great discovery. True cure must proceed from the center to the circumference, from above to below, from inward to outward, from the more important to the less important organs, from the head to the hands and to the feet. It is the homeopathic understanding that symptoms that move in this fashion go away permanently. When a symptom disappears in a reverse order of coming, the homeopath is sure that it is a true and lasting healing.

> ***If the external symptoms go first, it is a mere palliation; the disease is still remaining in the interior plane and is likely to occur again.***

If the physician believes that material changes in the body are things that disturb health and are the fundamental cause of the sickness, he may try to remove them surgically. By removing a tumor surgically, the disease is not gone. That which disturbed the physical economy is still in the body. It is subtle and cannot be removed by a surgical knife. Therefore, Hahnemann states in *Organon,* "The physician is a preserver of health if he knows the things that derange health and cause disease."[8]

Most people know now that the crude drugs administered by orthodox physicians in no way stimulate the healing responses; they only suppress and hide symptoms and give temporary relief. Since what causes disease is so subtle, is internal and operates from the center to the circumference, the drugs used must be of such quality to fight the disease. So, only a simple substance of the same electromagnetic resonance or vibrational level of the interior economy can stimulate the organism towards healing. The genius of homeopathy accomplishes it by the Law of Similars and potency. The word *potency* in homeopathy is defined as the energy of the medicine. Each potency is associated with a particular level of energy. The higher the potency, the greater is its intrinsic energy. This is an invisible subtle energy. You cannot test it in a lab, but it is clinically proven in a myriad of cases where it is properly applied.

Individuality and Symptoms

The Law of Similars demands that the doctor shall find correspondence and likeness between the patient's picture and the picture of remedy. When the individuality of the remedy corresponds to the individuality of the patient, only at that point does the remedy become homeopathic. In my understanding, hardly any medical discipline has taken the individuality of the patient as seriously as homeopathy. Homeopathy looks at the individual and not the disease. Each of us suffers a cold in his unique way, yet conventional medicine assumes that all colds are the same and administers a standard treatment. It offers a common group of drugs – one to dry the nose, another to reduce the cough, and still another to reduce the temperature. Homeopathy, on the other hand, looks for one remedy that will take care of all symptoms by stimulating the body's defense to fight the cold.

We cannot know one person from another unless each has some particular characteristic feature or expression that others do not show. Homeopathy observes sick people on this same principle observed in health, and thus it learns to individualize each patient.[9] The rare, peculiar, and strange symptoms in each individual reveal the clue to come to the right symptom, picture, and remedy. The ability to determine these strange, peculiar, and rare symptoms is a critical factor, which spells success in the homeopathic art. In homeopathy, taking a record of the patient is not a collection of facts. The homeopath is in the habit of studying the slightest shades of difference between patients, the little things that point to the remedy. Because of the little peculiarities manifested by every individual patient – through his inner life and through everything that he thinks, acts, and expresses – the homeopath is able to individualize the remedy. One needs intelligent observation to individualize medicine. The patient feels trust in the homeopath who pays personal attention to him. Response to treatment, dosage, and duration of treatment all are individualized. Every element works together to contribute maximum health to the patient without any side effects. It is almost impossible to have side effects, since the medicine has no atoms of the original drug. Homeopathy believes people get sick in individual ways showing distinctive patterns of symptoms. Homeopathy observes signs and symptoms in the mind, as well as in the body, before they allow tissue change or organ damage. If one waits for the end results, disease becomes incurable, and its true nature will be shrouded.

Homeopathic treatment is not aimed at treating the affected organs. It treats the person and not the affected organs. The remedy selected by the Law of Similars is designed to reach out to the root cause of the disturbance and to make the sick well again. It never injures the human organism by therapies. Its application and effect is gentle. It does not exhaust the patient's vitality. Rather, it stimulates the healing forces from within in a dynamic fashion making recovery rapid and safe.

Our anatomical individuality does not stop at faces and fingerprints. It extends to the whole internal anatomy. Therefore, homeopathy takes into account the physical appearance of the patient, too, when it administers constitutional medicine. Bodies differ in function as well as in form. People are biochemically unique. Biochemical individuality is one reason for variations in response to drugs.[10] The truth that everybody is different makes generalization risky about the benefits and hazards of foods and medical treatment. These days so many different diets are marketed and promoted as an antidote for obesity. I doubt there is such a right diet out there. A right diet probably exists differently for each individual. What is best for me need not be best for another person and might not even be best for me after a couple of years. The genius of homeopathy has realized this truth from its very beginning and, hence, individualized medicine.

Whenever there is a crisis in the system, the body tries to heal itself. This indicates action in the direction of healing. Symptoms and the resultant suffering are part of the body's endeavors to heal. Scientific medicine should heal people with minimum damage. But, scientific medicine is invasive and acts through means that involve destruction, inhibition, masking, and substitution. Most medicines carry an insert warning of the possible dangerous effects of the medicine. Homeopathic medicines neither destroy nor suppress the problem. They are stimulative in nature without toxic reactions. How homeopathic medicines work is not fully explained. In light of the discoveries of modern physics, it has now become much more intelligible. It is believed that the electromagnetic signals or energies are transferred in the diluted homeopathic preparations that retain the "memory" of the mother tincture, thereby triggering a response in the body.

We do not knowingly choose disease, but we make ourselves vulnerable by our surrender to medical theories, practices, and myths regarding health. Modern medicine heals millions of people. It also kills and injures millions. You need to make educated decisions sometimes regarding what treatments you need, what alternatives are available, and what treatments you have to decline. Sometimes the answers to our health problems are with us and around us. One just needs to know where to look.

8

Spirituality and Health

In the past two decades, I have had the opportunity and privilege to participate in the healing process of many patients suffering from various kinds of illness. Some of them were healed and some of them were not, as has been happening in all times. In some instances, I witnessed recoveries that cannot be fully explained by science. In my practice, I observed the power of one's religious faith acting as an instrument in recovery. I do not think I am an exception to have noticed such phenomenon. Many physicians have, I am sure, observed it. Most of them preferred to keep silent lest they should look less scientific. Scientific medicine is gingerly edging towards the acknowledgement of spiritual factors in health and healing. Doctors trained in Western medicine find it hard to accept faith as a factor in health and healing. The idea of including spirituality in the clinical card was something unimaginable.

Healing, ordinary or miraculous, enjoys a crucial role in the holy writings of almost all religions. The control of disease and maintaining health has been a concern in the religious expressions of humanity. In the early days of humanity, the spiritual priest and medicine man were one and the same. Healing was mainly a faith-based enterprise until the nineteenth century. Faith-based medicine then gave way to a more scientific medicine and its priesthood, the physician. The spiritual dimension of health was overlooked by the rational and empirical discipline. When experimental science and its measurements became an accepted standard of science, religion, rooted in intuition and subjective experience, was reduced in importance. Since empirical methods cannot be applied to religious experience and duplicated, the existence of God and the experience of God that involves religion, was looked down upon to be unscientific. Health professionals are now coming to know that a person's faith has a very strong influence over his health and well-being. This was ignored for some decades by orthodox medicine and is now being rediscovered by the science. Physicians trained in empirical science created a great divide between body, mind, and spirit. As a result, it lost touch with complementary methods that can help people heal.

Here, I refer to spirituality in a more inclusive manner. It is a broader concept than religion and is a dynamic, personal, and experiential process. The features of spirituality include a quest for meaning and purpose; an attitude and orientation to the Transcendent, or something larger than one's own self and material existence. Religious faith, rituals, and prayers are all different means to connect one with the Transcendent. Many patients have found greater health and well-being through prayer, worship, and by the support of the faith community.

Faith Has Positive Health Benefits

Surveys suggest that most patients have a spiritual life and regard their spiritual health just as important as their physical health. Oftentimes, people have greater spiritual needs in times of serious illness. Most studies have shown that religious involvement and spirituality are associated with better health outcomes, including longevity, coping skills, a better health-related quality of life, and less anxiety, depression and suicidal tendencies. Several studies have also shown that addressing the spiritual needs of the patient may actually enhance recovery from illness.

Generally speaking, ninety percent of people from all cultures believe in a Higher Being. A majority of the nearly three-hundred fifty studies that have examined physical health, and in the eight-hundred fifty studies examining mental health, that have considered religious and spiritual variables, have found that religious involvement and spirituality are associated with better health outcomes.[1] Many physicians question the appropriateness of addressing religious or spiritual issues within a medical environment. They feel religion is a sensitive and personal area too private for the physician to inquire about. If the physician sees that one's past physical history is important in diagnosis and treatment and has no problem in inquiring and eliciting information from the personal or private life of the patient, then the spiritual domain need not be seen as something inappropriate. The only governing factor is that the physician shall not impose his beliefs or be judgmental.

Physicians may not be competent to handle the spiritual needs of a patient, as is true with many physicians; in these cases, the referral method is the best way. Almost all hospitals in the West have spiritual caring facilities, with competent and trained personnel in the field of the respective religions. Physicians can make spiritual inquiry, without being intrusive, to see if the patient has any spiritual struggles, whether their faith can be used to cope with the stress of the illness. Sometimes one's belief system has to be taken into account in the medical decision-making process. It is encouraging to note that many health practitioners are serious about integrating body, mind, and spirit with the modern medical practice.

There is prolific and compelling evidence telling the vital role of spiritual practices on human health. The benefits of religious involvement have been well documented by scientific studies over the last few decades, studies published in authoritative medical journals such as the *American Journal of Public Health, The American Journal of Psychiatry, The American Journal of Medicine,* and many others. I would like to briefly summarize a few benefits underscored by such reputable journals, namely:

- Recovering faster and with fewer complications if you develop a serious illness.
- Encountering a life threatening and/or terminal illness with greater peacefulness and less pain.
- Avoiding mental problems like depression, anxiety and stress.
- Steering clear of problems, such as alcoholism, suicide, etc.
- Less fear of death and anxiety.
- Higher level of emotional well-being.

Because of the gaping chasm between medical science and religion, these beneficial elements have been woefully neglected.

In 1991, a study of 1,077 students at Northern Illinois University reported that the highly religious student had better overall health, less sickness, fewer doctor visits, and fewer injuries than their less-than-religious or non-religious friends.[2] Religion generally promotes healthier lifestyles, habits, and moral behaviors. These factors may not be the sole reason for better health. However, a healthy lifestyle alone cannot furnish a satisfactory explanation for this kind of positive impact on health. One's religious commitments are often expressed in external actions that are observable: abstaining from alcohol, tobacco, meat, etc. Apart from the observable healthy actions and practices, religious commitment itself is a very powerful means to open up the channels of healing energy into one's system.

The How and Why of the Faith Factor

Health benefits of faith are often a by-product of one's religious commitment. The goal of faith is to become close to the Creator and to discern God's plan and commit oneself to it. By doing so, one may get restored. Though religious involvement appears to decrease your chances of getting sick, it does not eliminate them. When serious illness strikes, religion seems to boost the recovery process significantly. A 1986 study in Virginia indicated that strong religious beliefs and its practice led to a significant impact in recovery.[3] People who have had a spiritual experience reported the benefits of the same relaxation response as mentioned earlier. It seems that religious involvement generates some kind of relaxation by its worship, aesthetics, fellowship, rituals, etc. Rituals of all kinds play a role in our daily life. They give us a sense of security and comfort. Our brains are designed to hold on to the experience of rituals. In every religion, there is a strong resistance to change rituals that have existed for a long time, even if their meaning has faded in the present context. When religious rituals are changed, people feel some discomfort and uneasiness. Obsessive-compulsive disorders are naïve endeavors of the mind to hang on to rituals that assure some sense of security.

> ***Faith is a potent weapon to bring about relaxation responses capable of restoring stressed-out organs.***

It is generally noticed that in life crises and challenges, people who can turn to spiritual sources and support cope more effectively and keep their sense of well-being.

In all probability, faith is a potent weapon to bring about relaxation responses in the body. When the mind is quieted, worries are lifted; stressed organs begin to restore themselves. This explanation does not limit religious involvement as a tool for relaxation. Besides the above experience, a good number of religious people have reported that an energy force envelops them, so much so, that they feel they are in touch with some life force that is restoring them. Although Western science does not acknowledge any subtle energy, nevertheless, almost all cultures universally have believed in some energy force to which you can connect yourself by intention and will.

Since the God experience is something subjective and cannot be easily measured by scientific standards, we can only depend on human experience and anecdote. Religion is a question of an inner journey where science has limited entry. Believers do not need any scientific data to validate their experience. Dr. Jeffrey S. Levin wrote in the *Journal of Social Science and Medicine*, "The mere belief that religion or God is health enhancing may be enough to produce salutary effects..." Various scriptures promise health and healing to the faithful, and the physiological effects of expectant beliefs such as this are now documented by mind-body researchers. Gospels emphatically have laid out the power of faith and its need for believers.

Faith in a nurturing, guiding, loving, and forgiving God can produce miraculous results in the human body because we are wired to believe. Belief in oneself, nature, medicine and other people – physicians and healers – are powerful to effect healing for certain types of illnesses. By the same token, belief in a Transcendent Power, who has the will and might to help us in need, can work to effect positive changes in the body. This is all the more powerful a belief than other beliefs in the hierarchy because holy writs, seers, saints, mystics, and the universal human experience support them. Therefore, faith can produce miracles.

Your religious beliefs are your spiritual muscles that can unleash certain mind-body mechanisms towards health and healing.

It is possible that sacred and divine experiences are accessible through various means other than religious involvement. Simple meditation without any religious imagery can bring people almost the same experience that can be drawn from religious meditation. Buddhist meditations for enlightenment do not have, strictly speaking, any religious qualities. Yet, they are capable of producing similar spiritual results. A November 28, 1994, *Newsweek* article reported that outside of attending church, forty-five percent of Americans sense the sacred during meditation, whereas sixty-eight percent have this sense at the birth of a child, and twenty-five percent during sex. This means the sacred and divine come to us through many channels and varied ways.[4]

In spite of our great strides in technology and science, our control of nature and its vagaries is limited. We do not control fifty percent of the events happening in our lives. None of us can solve all the problems of life, even with the best of intention and effort. People of faith are naturally taught to turn to God when life hurts and misfortunes hit. In faith, people look to their God for guidance, strength, and endurance. 'Let go and let God' is a powerful mantra. True religious faith acts out this mantra with a sense of surrender to the Transcendent. It helps one to acknowledge God's power and willingness to help and opens oneself to the healing love and energies from a different source.

The effect of religious commitment is primarily in the mind. From the mind, it naturally flows into the body. We already have discussed the role the mind plays in health and healing. Faith is a powerful emotional nourishment to the spirit, as food and exercise is to the body. Religion and its rituals remind us of the transcendent dimension of human existence, which helps to shift focus away from the daily cares and woes and invites us to communicate with a Holy One who has greater plans for us. Rituals can give us a sense of security as a way of connecting oneself to the Transcendent.

Religious commitment and faith teach us to hope. Religious traditions are a constant supply of hope. Hope is a dynamic factor that propels humans to expect good in the midst of apparent evil. The quality of hope has a boosting effect. Our brain rewires itself when it is fed with hope. Religious life and worship give a framework to set in motion the power of positive expectancy. It has a placebo effect. Remember our earlier discussion that more healings are made out of placebo effects than the actual effects of medicine. Placebos work for anyone simply because they believe they will. In religious commitment, there is something more than the placebo. Religious participation generally helps to alleviate stress by promoting optimism and hope.

Religious commitment and faith take one out of the present situation and shift the perspective to gain one's true identity and relationship with God. Truth has the power to liberate both mental and physical afflictions. Generally, religion promotes greater optimism and hope, irrespective of the quality relationship with the Transcendent.

Religious involvement and spiritual practices can promote positive emotions and limit the bad impact of negative emotions. We know how our body repairs itself and builds health by shifting to the parasympathetic branch of the autonomous nervous system when it is normal; that is, without fear, anxiety, hostility, and anger. The result is decreased blood pressure, heart rate, and oxygen consumption as against the sympathetic nervous system control time. So, religious involvement and spiritual practices can lead to psychological and physiological benefits. Compared with religiously uninvolved persons, religiously involved persons have an enhanced immune function. Religiously involved people enjoy a strong social support system; the physical and mental health benefits of such elements are well-known.

All religious traditions have emphasized the importance of loving God and neighbor. We look for the human experience of love in all our involvements. It is in love, and in the experience of being loved, that humans actualize their potential. People who help other people consistently report better health than their peers in the same age group. It has been observed that many people who do volunteer work out of altruism have improved their health markedly. Medications can alter the brain's balance of neurotransmitters and can lead to improvement in mood and overall function. Similar changes must be taking place in religious involvement.

It is estimated that twenty-five percent of hospital visits and medical reliance can be reduced by employing one's own resources. Religious faith and involvement are effective in areas of psychosomatic problems.

Psychosomatic diseases have their genesis in the mind. This in no way makes the condition, nor its problems and suffering, less real. Even though faith and beliefs have legitimate healing powers, healing through faith and belief is looked down upon by many. In a recent investigation of faith-healing in Baltimore, Maryland, sixty-seven percent claimed some positive effect on physiological problems, but greater results were recorded on the psychological level. Some of the medical problems that can be healed by spiritual or psychic healers are:

- Angina pectoris
- Bronchial asthma
- Ulcers, cold sores
- Backaches, abdominal pain, pain in the leg or arm
- Dizziness
- Impotency
- Insomnia
- Colds, coughs
- Constipation
- Deafness
- Skin reactions

Faith is no guarantee that these medical conditions can be influenced. Medical problems are often the result of a number of variables. However, once a malady strikes, the resources of faith can enhance the healing process. It helps lift the burden of the delimiting illness. Palliative medicine emphasizes psycho-spiritual and psychosocial aspects of care. Terminally ill patients report significantly greater religiousness facing death with the spiritual perspective compared with healthy people. A greater depth of the spiritual perspective is associated with a greater sense of well-being. Surveys suggest that religiously involved persons at the end of life are more accepting of death, unrelated to the belief in an after-life.[5] Religious involvement predicts greater functioning among disabled persons. Religious involvement is associated with fewer hospitalizations and shorter hospital stays.

Illness may interrupt routines, drain finances, separate families, create situations of dependency, and lead to existential and spiritual concerns. People who are religiously involved and spiritually active cope with these situations with a minimum impairment to their health system. Religious and spiritual coping are common among nursing home residents and elderly populations. Religious and spiritual coping have shown amazing results in dealing with HIV, asthma, skin burns, multiple sclerosis, chronic pain, etc. Religious and spiritual coping have been shown to buffer the noxious effects of stressful life events, such as the death of a spouse, divorce, etc.

One study examined the relationship between religious coping and depression among eight-hundred fifty men who had no history of mental illness and were hospitalized for a medical illness.[6] After adjustment for socio-demographic and baseline health variables, depressive symptoms were inversely related to religious coping. In addition, religious coping was the only baseline variable that predicted less depression six months later. Religious people are less likely to abuse alcohol and other drugs. More than twenty studies have been published on this particular issue. The inverse relationship between religious involvement and suicide was reported in a number of studies.

Faith seems to have more importance when one contracts severe illness. It gets them through hard times. They cope better with less anxiety and stress-related problems. In a recent survey, when asked how religious experiences had affected the way they dealt with illness, ninety-three percent of women said that religion helped them to sustain hope. Faith can boost the immune system. Researchers at the Duke University Medical Center took blood samples of 1,718 volunteers, age 65 or older, to look for chemicals associated with enhanced immunity. They found that the older adults who frequently attended religious services had slightly healthier immune systems.

Faith can boost the immune system. The brain rewires itself when it is fed with hope.

A study of forty heart transplant patients at the University of Pittsburgh Medical Center found that those with strong beliefs, who were involved in religious activities after their transplants, had better physical and emotional health.[7] The researchers made the discovery after asking the recipients about their faith and health at intervals of two, seven, and twelve months after their operations. Those who were more likely to report better physical health by the end of twelve months were patients who felt that their beliefs exerted greater influence over their lives and who consulted God to make important decisions. Not only that, but these same people found themselves to be less worried about their health. Authentic faith and religious involvement do not make health as a goal; it comes as a by-product of a true search for God, acknowledging God in good times and bad times equally.

Dr. David Larson, who conducted many studies in the field of religious involvement and health, remarked, "When people have severe illness where their lives are at risk, there is an increase in the role religion can play." The implications are that health professionals need to recognize the importance of the patient's religion or spirituality when dealing with such disease. Even though the survival rates of terminal illnesses are less impressive because of religious involvement or spiritual practices, nevertheless, it has lessened pain and promoted a sense of well-being.

Faith and Emotional Well-Being

Faith can help people living in slow pace or sometimes miraculously to regain better health when it is lost. The faith factor is a protective effect and also noteworthy. In a study that assessed the psychological health of the members of a Pentecostal Church in Newfoundland, it found that church members who participated more actively in church activities reported significantly fewer symptoms of psychological distress than those who participated less in such activities. People who are actively involved in their religious worship and activities (not nominal believers who participate in religious activities as a social involvement) are less likely to suffer from significant mental illness and anxiety. It is generally noted that faith makes a difference in the suicide rate. In a 1974 study of seven-hundred twenty people with suicidal feelings, researchers found that individuals reporting suicidal feelings were less likely than their non-suicidal peers to belong to a religious organization or to attend religious services.[8] The point is that religious faith and its genuine practice can play a positive role in maintaining psychological health.

Religious values and religious dispositions are good antidotes for depression and anxiety. Good pastoral counselors can make a tremendous difference in their depressed patients. In one survey, men with low levels of religiosity scored almost twice as high on the depression scale as their more religious counterparts. People with religious commitment reveal better psychological adjustment and fewer physical symptoms in the wake of catastrophic events.

Although the liberal media and our contemporary culture have often portrayed religious people as being repressed, sour-faced, and having no excitement of life, scientists are now finding that the opposite is true. In a 1988 published study of 1,150 individuals examining the effect of religious involvement, it revealed that religiously involved people have a significantly higher degree of overall health satisfaction. The participants were asked to rate their satisfaction with marriage, work, and community along with other overall satisfactions.[9] In a 1982 study of seven-hundred nineteen women, researchers found that religious commitment was the most reliable predictor of contentment among women. Women are said to be more religious by nature than men. One's perception of God and the way one relates to God has its impact on one's sense of well-being and health.

If we look at God as the All-Powerful person out there, who enjoys all power and acts arbitrarily according to His will, and we are simply creatures at His mercy looking for the occasional doling out of favors when we pressure Him, it will have a bad consequence on one's mental and physical well-being. If we conceive of God as a friend, a source of abundance to which we can connect ourselves to and can draw on at any time for anything, then we are likely to derive greater satisfaction and well-being. Over the years, a good amount of research has underscored the importance of religious belief and practice, particularly when accompanied by a profound personal spirituality that can ease the life-shattering effects of grief and help people adjust to their losses.

Contrary to the popular myth that religious people are more neurotic than non-religious, the more religiously active people are less neurotic. I do not overlook the fact that religion with its positive dimension does have some definite risks and possible negative effects when misused. Any area of potential good can be distorted and corrupted easily. The fundamentalist understanding of religion and its practices, accordingly, have always created problems and earned a bad reputation for religion. Though religion is for spiritual growth, it can inhibit growth and self-realization by adding unnecessary rules and regulations. In fact, all mystics and saints have outgrown their religion. Psychologically, they were beyond the barriers of their religion. Some people with psychotic illness experience religious delusions and use religious language to express their distress. In some cases, pathology is triggered by their religious understanding and moral values. Even in such cases, religion can be a positive factor when properly handled.

Religious Aesthetics and Health

The human appreciation of beauty is universal. Humans have a craving for aesthetic pleasure on a deeper level. Aesthetic experiences enrich personality, lift up and refresh people. It creates a sense of wonder and awe. When a person experiences wonder and awe, he is in the presence of the Transcendent mystery of the universe. Actually, worship is the result of this sense of wonder and awe. Religious art and rituals connect people to the deity, awakening the aesthetic self. Religious music and paintings are a powerful means to transport the soul to a different realm of experience. Music has been shown to have many therapeutic effects. Music can help improve the mobility of stroke, lift depression and anxiety, and lessen pain. Listening to music can reduce an elevated blood pressure and/or heart rate. Anyone can take advantage of music for relaxation without any professional guidance.

Sacred music, ancient or modern, seems to penetrate into the whole being of the person, carrying the message of God's glory and God's love deeper into our being. Sacred music and singing allows people to engage their whole selves – body, mind, and spirit – God, being the supreme beauty, truth, author of life, and all that we can imagine.

Spirituals tend to praise the object of all these virtues. Glorifying God is an important part of all spiritual tradition. Psalms are full of praises, a poetic outpouring of praises from the heart. Music easily puts you into the mode of praying, bringing yourself together free from distraction. For this reason, most spiritual traditions invoke music at the outset of their worship services.

Music stirs our memories. When we hear favorite music from a particularly happy time in our life, it lifts up the spirit, refreshing the neural connections associated with that sound. When I hear old carol songs, I relive my childhood days when I joined the carol group going around to neighborhood homes singing, dancing, and having fun. Music and worship activate and unite us with other members of the community. It allows for many occasions to interact with others and increases a sense of common bond among believers. Numerous factors involved in religious worship and its practices invigorate the body, mind, and spirit.

Religion and Longevity

Humans cannot avoid death. It is part of being human. A number of factors are at play regarding human longevity. Researchers have found that gender, ethnicity, education, health status, degree of social support, etc., have their role in human health and longevity. Sociological studies have found that social isolation and lack of family support and care can raise the mortality rate higher. Lower mortality rates are seen among those who had frequent contacts with friends, relatives, religious support groups or associations.[10] In another study made on members of religious Kibbutzim and non-religious Kibbutzim, a notable difference was observed in the longevity of life. They had the same lifestyle, social structure, and family support systems. The only variable factor was religious observance, which made a fifty percent difference in the mortality rate.[11] Religiously involved people suffer less from fear of death and anxiety than non-religious people, according to a number of research studies. Religious involvement helps decrease the mortality rate in older individuals facing stressful events. Patients with life-threatening illnesses who kept their faith alive have been found to exhibit higher levels of emotional well-being and recovery.

Many studies have found that religious involvement aids people in coping with a variety of crises, boosting resilience, peace of mind, and endurance. Dying patients with strong religious beliefs reported significantly lower levels of death anxiety than their non-religious counterparts, a 1978 study testifies.[12] Human beings under the threat of imminent death reflexively reach for the comfort and sustenance faith offers.

Breaking Addictions

Nowhere in medicine has religious involvement and spiritual practices shown more influence than in the field of addiction recovery. Science has shown faith resources to be critically important in preventing and treating substance abuse and addictive behavior. Addicted people have a great and real dependence on substances as they use them. Addictions to alcohol, tobacco, and cocaine are still difficult to treat successfully. But, the faith factor can make a difference in these kinds of disorders. When dependency is weaned slowly, the individual needs something, or someone, to lean on in order to fill the void. Faith and trust in a benevolent God fill this vacuum. Many people who are successful in killing addictions have reported the spiritual component of the recovery as a major factor in regaining and maintaining sobriety.

Alcoholism expert Dr. William Miller remarked, "Alcoholism drives out spirituality and spirituality drives out alcoholism." It seems that the vacuum caused by the absence of religious involvement is too often filled by alcohol or drug abuse. The spiritual practice that is helping scores of alcoholics to achieve and maintain sobriety is not based on one's willpower, but surrender to a "Higher Power." Their way of gaining control over the substance is letting go of their control and letting God control by a loving surrender.

In a 1991 study of alcoholics and drug addicts, researchers found that alcoholics who had achieved long-term sobriety had developed spiritual practices in conjunction with their Alcoholics Anonymous (AA) participation.[13] Almost one-hundred percent of them said they meditated or prayed daily. Complete recovery is frequently accompanied by profound spiritual change and conviction. Psychiatrist Gerald May remarked, "Any sincere battle with a particular addiction is likely to bring us to some kind of spiritual confrontation, and any spiritual journey is certain to involve very practical struggles with addiction."

The twelve-step program of AA provides a therapeutic community for alcoholic recovery. It gives support and structure to overcome addiction as AA extends a network of caring people who share their commitment to sobriety. AA is a caring religious community, though it has no formal religious affiliation or any formal practice of religion. It is different from a traditional religious community, but at the same time, it provides all the advantages of a religious group. It even has a scripture, *The Big Book of Alcoholics Anonymous*. It has set rituals, specific ways of relating to each other, and relating to God. It shares common wisdom and supports one another as sponsors and friends. It acts as a therapeutic group, above all encouraging the expression of feelings to help assess one's proper role without inducing guilt. Sometimes it confronts lovingly. In numerous ways, AA provides structure and accountability to help the alcoholic build a new life that is not centered on drinking. The absence of a sense of purpose and direction makes a feeling of emptiness in life. AA gives their members a sense of purpose and rootedness through spiritual commitment. Helping each other, they lift up their own spirits as well as others. Doing good for fellow humans uplifts the giver and the receiver.

Prayer and Its Benefits

People of all faith believe in the power of prayer. Atheists will reject the power of anything spiritual. Believers do not need medical proof for the power of prayer. The evidence is simply overwhelming. They might even think it as blasphemous to subject faith and prayer to the lab of scientists, for it is like testing God and God's power. But it need not be seen that way. When something affects the human body, it becomes a legitimate concern of medicine to find out more about it so that it can be applied to more people and to promote the benefit of it to a larger section of the society. In fact, it has already happened. So many investigative studies of late have proven this fact conclusively.

Prayer is the natural outcome of the human heart to the Transcendent when it acknowledges that the reason for its existence is outside of itself. If I have not created my life nor control it fully and take it to its destiny or final fulfillment, then naturally, I am inclined to lean on that Force or Power that sustains me and guides me through life to its destiny. Prayerfulness is the result of the recognition that the Power outside me is willing to help me and has the power to do so. The awareness of this Power is inherent in humans, or as we say, it is natural. Science simply now tells us that relating to this Transcendent Power has many health benefits. Science is not concerned about the nature of the Transcendent nor its purpose to bring healing.

To seek the meaning of illness or health is outside the purview of science. Nonetheless, science agrees when people pray, they effect some changes in their mind and body. Conversation with God is not limited to any religious tradition, although religious traditions may help to do it in an effective way in most instances. Prayer is one of the known ways to communicate with the Transcendent. God will naturally work in the life of humans who confide in His power and goodness. It can be direct or indirect. Direct intervention of God is rare, though its evidence has not been fully rejected. When it happens, we say a miracle has occurred.

Most cures obtained through prayer are by indirect means. God has many agents and assistants – nature, medicine, doctors, etc. God works in us, with us, among us. Knowledge of pharmaceuticals, surgery, psychology, and other conventional and non-conventional methods of treatment are all gifts from God.

> ***It is foolish and irresponsible not to combine the best physical, psychological, and spiritual care available.***

We, as humans, have a tendency to view God in certain compartments of life, and in other compartments of life, God is fully absent. First, one has to recognize that all healing comes from God. There is no single way to be healed. There is no special time to be healed. If you are obese, healing comes when you change your diet, start exercising, and remove the emotional barriers.

Healing is a natural part of our human condition and a gift from the Creator. God's timing may not match our desires, but prayer speeds healing. Prayer contains the greatest coping mechanism, as we have noted earlier. Whether or not you receive what you ask for in the manner you want, one thing is sure: prayer will change you. You are changed when you pray; that in itself will be the precious outcome of prayer. In the classical spiritual traditions and writings, it says that prayer does not change God or God's will; but it changes your attitudes, values, perspectives, etc. These changes eventually help some to find a cure.

People who trust in God learn the art of trusting in God and letting go. It is by this 'letting-go' attitude that healing often takes place. Prayer is not intended to pressure God to heal us but to accept God and life as they are, thereby allowing the spiritual energies to flow freely in life and heal us. Do not challenge God by defining exactly how you expect a healing to take place. One may wonder what kinds of prayers are most likely to be heard. Scientific research seems to be finding that it is the prayers we truly believe in, the ones in which we invest our deepest emotions and our strongest desires, regardless of how we choose to voice our prayers. Larry Dossey, the author of *Healing Words,* examined more than one-hundred thirty studies of prayer effectiveness and came to the conclusion that all forms of prayer work, but non-directed prayer may have a slight edge over other forms. This is the "Thy Will Be Done" form of prayer.

Prayer in its inclusive definition is simply a state of being with God by reverence, adoration, meditation, atonement or vocal praying. Prayer belongs to all God's children, irrespective of religion and religious denominations, and is likely to be answered with no strings attached. Herbert Benson, a top medical scientist and president of the Mind/Body Medical Institute, reports that when a patient is wired to machines that monitor brain waves, blood chemistry, heart rate, stress levels, etc., and is asked to pray, changes have taken place in the level of cortisol, epinephrine, and norepinephrine. These are hormones that compromise the immune system and increase our likelihood of developing heart disease, stroke, ulcers, and many other stress-related diseases.

Healing does not always mean a complete physical cure. Prayer brings healing always. The beauty and power of prayer is that you can have a sense of healing even when physical integrity is lacking. Healing must be looked upon in a much broader way than miraculous changes in one's body. Whether or not the desired cure takes place, healing is available to all who genuinely pray. Larry Dossey believes that not to employ prayer with patients is equivalent of deliberately withholding a potent drug or surgical procedure. He found in many experiments that a simple attitude of prayerfulness seemed to set the stage for healing. The fact that prayer works tells us something about our human nature. We are spirit-incarnated in our bodies and we have a natural connection to the world of spirit. By connecting oneself to the source of one's existence, one can find a sense of meaning, purpose, and well-being.

Since humans do not control the spiritual and the Transcendent, neither can they dictate to it; the only possible thing is to have openness to accept and receive God's communication and action through varied channels and means. Since God's ways are not fully known to humans, they do not follow a consistent pattern as we humans would like it to be (God being God, God's freedom for the infinite and varied ways of working is not limited by any means we can imagine). Prayer effects cannot be duplicated in the lab context like other experiments. Variables affect the research in different degrees. When variables are related to a different domain, such as the spiritual and transcendent, it is almost impossible to apply strict scientific rules. Prayer by its very nature transcends time and space; therefore, it belongs to the transcendental realm.

Finite humans may not be able to handle and apply a transcendental reality to mere earthly purposes and plans. It should be employed with its overall purpose of life on earth. The efficacy of healing prayers, I believe, is dependent on the ultimate meaning and goals of life. It is more the totality of life that is probably considered in the granting of our prayers. That means the efficacy of prayer would sometimes be miraculous, sometimes slow, and sometimes non-existent. By the same token, strictly speaking, prayer does not belong to the lab experiment. How faith or prayer works in promoting health is less measurable than other factors that can be easily measured. (To demonstrate causality in medical research, a finding must be consistent and replicable). There is no individual medicine that can produce exactly the same results in two people. When it comes to faith, things are still more complicated. We will never fully know how the faith factor works because the transcendental dimension of life does not yield all of its secrets at once.

Whatever is not measurable and duplicated does not enjoy validity in the scientific world. One's commitment to prayer, its intensity and right dispositions – all these are very subjective and cannot be quantified and measured in determining the effect of prayer offered for healing. This may be the reason that scientists were not interested to conduct studies in the field of prayer and health until recently. From a number of daring studies, the association between religious involvement and spirituality and better health outcomes seems valid. Nevertheless, not all mechanisms by which religious involvement and spirituality affect health are understood. Prayer does not require science to validate it.[14] But, in a culture where science is valued as the ultimate arbiter of what is real and what is illusion or unreal, if science says something positive about prayer, it may help many to employ this potent force in a more valuable manner in health and healing. Those who already believe in prayer may feel empowered in their convictions.

The effect of faith on human health can, to some extent, be measured but it cannot be fully controlled or understood. No one can plumb the depth of God's work and plan in human nature. We can still learn about it and can come to reasonable conclusions. Dale Matthews, who did extensive research and studies in the field says, "Faith is a unique combination agent that efficiently delivers a series of powerful interrelated ingredients promoting health and well-being."[15]

Extrinsic and Intrinsic Religion

Gordon Allport and J. Michael Ross, who made a study on the religious orientations of people, found there are two types of religious orientation; namely, extrinsic and intrinsic.[16] Extrinsic religion is a means to obtain another end such as health, security, power, etc. One may or may not be consciously aware of these ulterior motives. For them, secondary gains of religious involvement matter more than the essence of religious teachings. Such people may present convincing facades of religiosity. They may be regulars to the church and will accept all regulations of their church. They are usually seen as good supporters of the community to which they belong. Often these people are most vocal, reciting scriptures or doctrines to support their views in a given situation. Though these people work hard fulfilling the more visible and measurable requirements of their religious tradition, their hearts are not deeply engaged in a relationship with God. Their source of strength is not from their personal understanding and relationship with God, but rather from their unconscious psychological needs. Allport remarks that the extrinsic people, despite their apparent pro-religious stance, are likely to show more intolerance, prejudice, and hate than intrinsic religious people.

Intrinsically religious people care less about social conformities than do their extrinsic brothers and sisters. These more authentic religious people are likely to receive health benefits from religious involvement than those with extrinsic orientation. Intrinsic people are often found doing the thankless and unglamorous work in the religious communities. Intrinsic people follow a more disciplined devotional life characterized by humility and gentleness. They are less talkative about religion and spirituality but can guide other people by their religious experience. Extrinsic people use religion as a tool to gain their secular ends; they are less likely to draw the benefits of health by their religiosity.

A study in 1991 assessing the role of extrinsic and intrinsic religiosity in depression found that depression levels went up among people who scored high as being extrinsic on an inventory of religiosity traits.[17] This indicates that people who are deeply and authentically religious ward off depression more effectively than their counterparts.

The negative potential of religion has been very visible throughout history. Hatred, violence, social prejudice, and numerous wars have occurred in the name of religion. It is sometimes a two-edged sword. The positive potential of religion can hardly be overstated despite all the negatives recorded in its history. It is the same religion that has inspired millions of people to be generous, kind, compassionate, loving, cooperative and has given meaning to life while helping many cope with their illness and improve their health conditions.

The twenty-first century is witnessing some of the greatest medical breakthroughs regarding the health benefits of religiosity. Earlier scientists who took the faith factor seriously risked being labeled unscientific. They lost prestigious appointments. Researchers who have established faith factor benefits to health have forged ahead despite opposition. The medical effects of religion are not just a matter of faith, but now, also a matter of science. It is an area that deserves more attention and research.

9

The Mysterious and Deeper Dimension of Health

We have seen the potential of religiosity to enhance human health and a sense of well-being. When becoming ill, many people tend to become spiritual. A spirituality emerging from within may heal sickness, rather than a drug applied from the outside. Normally, most people have a tendency to accord wisdom to someone or something outside of oneself who promises healing. As we focus on outside help, internal healing powers lay dormant. The impulse to do something to alleviate pain and discomfort is understandable. And sometimes it is lifesaving. In humans, exteriority and interiority must be balanced. One must look inward, wonder, and ask questions from a different angle.

All people who experience health problems desperately look for healing. They go to different therapists, healers, and spiritual centers. At times, they fight and struggle too hard in order to be healed.

Despite the good efforts of the patient and the healer, sometimes no healing occurs. Who can explain why the same treatment will cure one person but not another? A probable hypothesis can be stated at times. Sometimes, an ill person goes to an outright fraud, and the ill person's faith heals him. Likewise, a good person goes to a devoted and sincere healer, and the patient remains as sick as he was before. I have noticed people becoming sick, and being healed, where physical explanations are insufficient or obsolete. Healing is not a question of feeling free from symptoms. It has a much deeper meaning and purpose.

Spiritual Healing

Most people who have had a healing experience credit their faith in God as the core of their strength and ability to heal themselves. Spirituality encourages faith that is directed toward God within them, so that the individual can explore the creative capacity of his own spirit. Authentic spirituality is the practice of honoring our relationship to God, to empower us further to cope with life. To heal the self is to transcend the self. Genuine healing cannot be limited to the mental or physical level. Healing will remain incomplete unless the human aspiration for transcendence is taken into account. According to Carl Jung, healing comes only from that which leads the patient beyond himself, and beyond his entanglement with the ego.[1] An opening of the internal doors of perception is required, however, to see the domain of the spirit infused in all aspects of material life. A radical separation between the natural and the spiritual exists only in the unenlightened situation. Spiritual healing occurs through the attainment of the transcendent self. This state will free oneself from internal conflicts and suffering.

It is the experience of many that prayer works. The evidence is simply overwhelming, as we have previously noted. But does it always help? Absolutely not! Who can explain that prayer heals some diseases at times when the doctors and medicines have not been able to heal? Since prayer belongs to the transcendental realm, we cannot understand, with our ordinary perception, why some prayers are heard and some are not. As in the case of medicine, prayer does not work at all times. Without referring to the meaning and purpose of life, health and healing may not be fully understood. Treating a bacterial infection with penicillin is very effective in bringing about a cure. But, if it is applied to a viral infection, it will not be effective at all. It is not the failure of the medicine, but rather the application of it in the right context. Prayer fails because it is not properly applied contextually. Though humans can have some knowledge about how and when prayer could be more effective, humans do not possess the knowledge that predicts the outcome succinctly. This is part of our human limitation, rather than the limitation of the tool.

Being spiritual or holy is no guarantee for good health. Bad health or illness does not imply any spiritual sickness. In fact, many holy persons and spiritual giants had long struggles with illness. Most saints and mystics seemed to accept illness as part of the natural order. I believe they experienced healing of a different kind: a psychological healing which enabled them to accept the discomforts and pains of illness with serenity and gentleness. Our understanding of the relationship between spirituality and healing is vastly incomplete. It is a mystery and essentially something beyond human understanding. I believe the suffering saints and seers experienced a higher degree of health, though their physical bodies were breaking down. Health and illness paradoxically coexisted in them.

Sometimes illness is the only time people look upward and inward, and develop an appreciation for the transpersonal nature of their struggles.

People who experience a higher degree of health will have a sense of gratitude and contentment about life, despite the sickness. Ill health is not always negative. Illness can be an important opportunity to reflect upon one's life, and to set new priorities and values. Sometimes it is the only time people look upward and inward. Most lives go unexamined due to the hectic pace of everyday life. As the result of illness, many have learned to look at the world, God, and people in a totally different way. When you let go of your ego-level attachments and connect yourself with the spiritual and transcendent, your world is expanded. You move out of the individual pathology and suffering, and develop an appreciation for the transpersonal nature of your struggles. Then, what you are dealing with is not merely illness, but an awareness of your anguish or suffering that acquires a new meaning for you and the world. With this new awareness, the body is brought into a greater synchronicity and harmony with nature, with or without illness.

The art of creating purpose in life decides the tempo of human lives. Without finding a meaning or goal in life, humans cannot function optimally. Nutrients, exercise, and the right food all help to build health and healing; but without an accompanying sense of deeper purpose in life, long-standing health is difficult to attain. Our genes and brains have evolved to crave for meaning in life. One may be an avowed agnostic or atheist, but his mind and brain resists it because it has evolved into seeking a soothing and healing faith in a benevolent God. Many who meet with illness and catastrophes have embraced religion and faith, which they once disregarded. Nothing makes God more real to people than the prospect of illness and death. The capacity for faith in the power of a healing God is uniquely implanted in humans. Naturally, humans look to God for health and wholeness. In nearly all cultures prayer, religious rituals, and meditations have been used to find relief and healing from bodily and spiritual stress.

Humans often overlook their spiritual essence, or self, due to ego identification. Ego keeps drawing attention to itself, preventing one from looking into the inner self. It is that part of us that is connected to all humanity and to all life. As long as the ego has its grip on us, the inner self is not able to guide us towards our destiny. It is the transcendent or spiritual self that holds the power to heal. One might look at this wisdom first before one tries to pray or medicate it away. Even the willingness to experience pain and the acceptance of unpleasantness can transform one into something different.

The idea that bliss and happiness automatically come to us as we achieve our unity with the Universal self is highly popular. However, it is oftentimes misleading. We need the willingness to stand in the midst of mystery, to tolerate the ambiguity and the unknown, as part of the work towards healing.[2] This does not mean accepting disease passively. In the face of suffering, death, or misfortune, healing may not be possible until we learn to accept what cannot be changed, and remain open to our experience without the judgment of fault or virtue added to it.

The Unique Human Nature

Human beings are unique though they share one common human nature. We may share a Collective Unconscious awareness and have the same innermost desires and longings. Beyond that, every human is an individual with a specific anatomical makeup. No two people have the same kind of stomach and heart pattern. Variations in the branching of coronary arteries determine the chances of surviving heart attacks. So, it is presumable that individual difference is one factor that renders people susceptible to a particular disease.

Some individual differences help certain people to make a speedy recovery. People are biochemically unique. As much as individuals are unique, health benefits from herbs, food, and treatment will have a different impact on different people. Smoking cigarettes can cause cancer. But, it does not happen in the case of all individuals who smoke. Some may have a strong respiratory system that makes them immune from the bad effects of smoking, or their constitution is less susceptible to the cancerous virus. Medical benefits and hazards cannot be generalized.

For each individual, there may be a wide variety of possible responses to a disturbance. Some people are relatively unaffected by external or internal disturbances. People vary in their reaction to environmental influences. Some people are able to maintain a steady health, even with minimum hours of sleep, overwork, an erratic diet, and shouldering stressful responsibilities. For other people, if something more is added to their daily routine, they become stressed and suffer a variety of symptoms. While some people rarely notice heat or cold, others are very sensitive to it. The disturbances on health, thus, manifest themselves in a highly individualistic and varied manner.

Most naturopaths and nutritionists have contradicting arguments over the right way of healthful eating. There is no right way to eat healthily. The right diet for each individual can be found out only by observation and sometimes by the trial-and-error method. Ignoring individual differences, as well as generalizing from one's own experiences or experience with a few individuals, has led to contradictory dogmas about the health benefits of certain health practices, food, herbs, etc.

A perfect dietary medication for you should take into account your individual differences.

In a good number of cases, medical science works with probabilities. We know the disease-making factors, such as high cholesterol, high blood pressure, diabetes, smoking, lack of exercise, and heredity make the development of coronary disease more probable. However, it is difficult to say that every person who is subject to any one or more of these factors will develop a heart problem. Although medical science has made great strides in the past, our scientific knowledge of human health is by no means perfect.

The Potent Unconscious

It is the great discovery of psychology that most of our actions, reactions, responses, and attitudes originate from our unconscious. The vast majority of psychic life is not in the conscious mind, but in the unconscious. If this is the case, the conscious mind itself cannot create health and healing. Jung viewed the unconscious differently than Freud. To Freud, the unconscious was the seat of all uncontrollable, undesirable thoughts and desires. It is the seat of the id that is preoccupied with maximum pleasure and minimum discomfort. The goal of therapy is to tame the unconscious forces and bring them to conscious awareness. In contrast, Jung viewed the unconscious as the seat of archetypes and wisdom. This unconscious can be likened to a great reservoir where opposite forces wrestle to get the upper hand. He assumed that every psychic force has its counterforce in the unconscious – good with evil, darkness with light, love with hate, sickness with health, and so on. Health and wholeness are achieved by a dynamic balance of the innate opposites, and by making this balancing process as conscious as possible.

The unconscious, I believe, is the seat of our spiritual drives. Its potential is more powerful than our conscious drives. The unconscious is capable of violating the values of the conscious mind to achieve its ends. Therefore, sometimes it invokes illness, and sometimes it cures miraculously. It can violate known rules and conduct. Only those who move from the periphery of life will be able to understand the purpose and patterns of the unconscious. Sometimes, the unconscious reveals its goals and purposes through dreams, insight, intuition, etc. It has been shown that where the conscious mind lets go of its hold on our life and gives space to the unconscious, honoring its capabilities, one is most likely to receive greater health benefits.[3] Religiosity and prayer, by their very nature, help to let go of one's control in order to submit oneself to a higher wisdom. When people let go of their desperate need for healing, there arises a quality of acceptance and gratitude in spite of the disease. It is in such a state that miracles happen!

The unconscious is whispering to us in silence through visions, spiritual experiences, and insight. These visions, experiences, and insight can change our physical, mental, and spiritual faculties, and can alter our experience of the world. Most diseases are psychosomatic in their origin. Faith can help to heal psychosomatic diseases. Faith heals emotional wounds and promotes a catharsis by prayers, rituals, atonement, and forgiveness. As the result of that process, illnesses sometimes disappear.

Letting go of the conscious mind's control does not mean one should forgo surgery, medication, or other medical intervention that can be decidedly helpful. The underlying desire for total control of life, without any room for mystery and transcendence, is narcissism. It is only when the myth of self-sufficiency is shattered that the unconscious is experienced with its manifold blessings. If we pray and act only for what is acceptable to the conscious mind – less pain and discomfort

– we may be violating the wishes of the unconscious and its potent healing effects.

Almost all of us believe in the power of medicine to heal and restore health, although not all of the time. We know that faith and prayer can heal. Long before scientific medicine came into being, people became sick and were healed. Medicine can heal, and faith in a benevolent God, too, can heal. A combination of faith and medical resources can render a far greater health benefit, with healing being the natural outcome.

No Formulas

We cannot extract a formula or method for healing. No one formula works all of the time. A medicine that is capable of fully restoring health in some patients, fails to work in other patients. Medicine and surgery may work one-hundred percent of the time in some patients, but may show only a seventy-five percent or fifty percent success rate in others. It does not mean that the applied medicine is a failure. So many subjective elements are at work in any given healing. The interactive results of subjective and objective elements are beyond prediction. The lack of a precise measurement and prediction does not rule out the efficacy of medicine or the faith factor.

Neither faith nor medicine is a panacea against illness and death. Humans are human and, as such, mortality is part of our very nature. Most humans eventually die as the result of a short-term or long-term illness, if not by some accident, natural disaster, or catastrophe. The mortality rate of a human being has always been one hundred percent. It is often difficult to prove if it was God who healed or the medical treatment. Medical treatment is one modality of healing. Ultimately, any modality is also from God. A total absence or presence of faith, in itself, need not cause a disease or create a disease. No doubt, there are so many non-religious people who enjoy good health and longevity. So too, many deeply-devoted people get sick and sometimes are found struggling with terminal illness. Faith is one factor out of many factors in the complex web of health. It is the net result of so many factors interacting on a dynamic field. Health, though to some extent measurable, cannot be fully understood.

Sometimes healing comes to us quite miraculously by the direct intervention of God or the Transcendent. Oftentimes, healing comes slowly through the intervention of medical science and technology. God heals a person without the intervention of other people. But most often, God uses other people to participate in the healing; they may be healthcare providers, researchers, pharmacists, psychologists, pastors, etc. God has uniquely gifted people to participate in the healing process.[4] God's hand reaches out to us in manifold ways to heal us. Whether or not a desired cure takes place, as I mentioned in the beginning, healing is available to all of us.

People who have a genuine understanding of healing can accept healing on all three levels.[5] First, they understand the role of healing through medical science. Second, they accept the mystery of God's choosing to heal through non-medical ways. Third, they accept that, with all their good efforts and good intentions, they may not recover physically from illness and are not threatened by that possibility.

Ultimately, all healing is spiritual in nature. All the different names healers commonly refer to as their source of healing – Higher Consciousness, Super Consciousness, Infinite, Absolute, Universal Mind, Vital Force, Universal Energy – indicate that healing is not purely a matter of the human domain. Samuel Hahnemann, the founder of homeopathy, in the classical book *Organon Medicine*, states: "The more subtle the drug, the higher its curative power." The principle of the dilution remedy in homeopathy indicates that it is not any physical quality inherent in the substance that brings healing, but its spiritual quality – the subtle energy and the information it contains.[6] This is an indication that healing is spiritual in nature.

We, as humans, create our realities aided by the Transcendent. So, healing belongs both to the human and the divine realm. In our earlier surveys, we noted that our relationship with God by means of prayer, meditation, and meaningful rituals can positively affect high blood pressure, anxiety, wounds, and heart attack. These findings have been clearly brought out from numerous studies and experiments in the past. In dealing with health, we cannot overlook the role of one's religious faith and values. We are made to think that one must either choose the logical, analytical, and rational approach or the irrational, superstitious, and religious belief. From an unbiased perspective, one can no longer hold on to this attitude.

Science and spirituality can stand side-by-side in a complementary way to heal without eliminating each other.

There are many unforeseeable and unpredictable elements operative in the human health realm that give oneself reason to be optimistic beyond the use of any statistics. If the patient has a belief in prayer, encourage him to do so. Sometimes, the patient believes in certain rituals to bring healing. It may or may not be scientific and often may be superstitious. In the mysterious health realm, allowing the patient a chance to give his intuition a chance could bring out certain life forces or human potential. In every myth, there is some element of truth. What we discard as superstitious in the field of medicine may have redeeming factors that are not capable of being grasped or seen in such a situation.

We live in the world. It is equally true that the world lives in us. We are a microcosm of the world. Body and mind sound different and separate. Yet, they are indivisible and governed by an Intelligent Self. This intelligence can express itself in various ways. It sometimes expresses its purpose through illness, other times by healing. *What* is expressed is more important than *how* it is expressed. As Deepak Chopra puts it, "Health and disease are connected like variations of one melody, disease is a wrong variation." Most often, diseases are messengers to correct our values and functional modes to strike a greater balance in life. People hardly find time for self-exploration and examination or a reflective self-experience. So, one needs a disease or some stress to pull one out of one's rush-rush life. Diseases are sometimes triggered by our system's intelligence so that we may reach an optimum actualized life.

Afterword

Probably you will never hear a doctor ask the patient, "Are you a believer? Are you happy? Are you lonely, depressed, or unhappy?" Most doctors do not ask such questions. They fear it will make them appear less scientific. The scientific doctor does not understand that he can engender optimism and hope by promoting the patient's religious faith, which in turn would kick off his own healing mechanism. Doctors tend to look for hard proof for everything other than the orthodox treatment. There are events and phenomena that are not easily explainable by science. The scientific tunnel vision of allopathy sometimes prevents doctors from accepting a different medical tradition. Daring not to explore the possibilities of other forms of medicine with an open mind is a great disservice to humanity. Wisdom is not found in one culture, tradition, or philosophy, however perfect the claim of its proponents.

It is Samuel Hahnemann, the founder of homeopathy, who coined the word *allopathy*. It means 'other than the disease'. It was a denigrative word to describe orthodox medicine, because he thought it prescribed treatments on the basis of no logical or consistent relationship to symptoms. Allopaths disowned the name given to them, but somehow it slowly stuck to them. Then, later they came up with a new etymology from a German root meaning "all therapies", and claimed the system embraced all methods of proven value in the treatment of disease. The truth is that most allopaths do not live up to this new ideal of their redefined name. Some are very quick to condemn any other methods.

Medical science's belief that consciousness is a by-product of matter, and has no existence apart from matter, is a handicapped worldview. Belief in the primacy of matter is a cultural belief cultivated over the centuries. It is like any other myth. In order to have a therapeutic effect, there must be input on the material level, which is the basic philosophy of medical science. The primacy of consciousness over matter will challenge most of the medical notions prevailing today.

Energy is not a physical or material phenomenon, nor is it easily manipulated by ego-oriented intention. Medical science lacks a worldview that acknowledges subtle energy and consciousness in humans. There is a cultural bias to accept anything that is not material. Chinese acupuncture, based on the movement of Chi energy, is employed for anesthetic purpose and for many other ailments. Science views it suspiciously. Seeing its efficacy in treating certain ailments, medical scientists continue to search for a physical explanation for it. It was not ready to accept subtle energy movements and reorganization of disrupted energies in the human system. Deepak Chopra, the holistic health practitioner, aptly called this attitude "the superstition of materialism."

Conventional medicine presupposes that the ultimate cause of what happens is on the physical realm. It is part of a belief system that has no support. A science that defends and preserves its beliefs and refuses to be open-minded cannot be fully depended upon for authentic healing.

Education is the primary activity of the doctor and medicine. Often, doctors mystify things rather than clarify them to the patients so that they may be empowered. Knowledge is strength. This mystification may help financially and give some extra security to the doctors. However, prevention and management of disease is possible by methods less costly, dangerous, and more effective than what is practiced today, if true education and demystification of medicine occurs. People will learn to observe their bodies and should learn normal patterns of change, recognize early signs and symptoms of illness, and experiment with simple methods of treatment. Often, the only option people know is to surrender to conventional medicine and its authority. This surrender is surrendering to the disease.

Medical costs are soaring in most countries of the world. Preventive models are to be explored more vigorously. Learning more about the true cause of disease, and teaching people about how to recognize and manage it in the early stages, is critical in the management of disease. You have much more potential at your disposal than allopathy proposes. We have explored many of these alternatives in the earlier chapters.

In most holistic therapies, consciousness is considered as key to health and healing. This sometimes gives an occasional advantage over regular medicine, which disregards consciousness. Attitudes, values, and perspectives shape the way energy is organized and mobilized in our bodies. Using pharmaceutical drugs to influence biochemical and metabolic reactions is superficial and limited. Nature's medicines, instead of disrupting or diverting the chemistry of metabolism, convey complex informational patterns directly from nature to bring harmony and rhythm, with the flux and flow of the larger picture of which you are a part.

A wise healer employs what works. If the patient's worldview and beliefs are of a positive note, even if it may be in conflict with the therapist's view, it should be given a chance. Physicians should cultivate tolerance and flexibility in their approaches. If a patient has belief in prayer, chants, or herbs, let it be. There is a time for that. There is a time, too, when you can allow only for a scientific approach. If the belief of the patient and doctor coincide, it is most ideal and brings out the best. Conflicting beliefs may set the stage for disaster.

It is of great significance, if possible, to choose doctors who share your worldview. Most often, patients are attentive to the doctor's credentials, his specialties, training, and experience. Rarely do people think or explore the doctor's belief and worldview that could affect the therapy. What is commonly seen is surrendering to a doctor in the beginning, and then beginning to doubt and question the doctor's attitudes and values. If your surrender is total, it might help. If your worldview is in conflict with the doctor, it will adversely affect the therapy.

Patients sometimes accept medicines or go to the clinics not because they want to, but because someone pushes them. To please their family or household, they abide by certain medical practices. All of us are conditioned to think that medicine works and can cure you if you take it into your body. As we discussed earlier, faith itself is medicinal and often more powerful than the medicines' ability to heal.

There is a lot of bad research out there in the name of scientific medicine. Medical journals are cluttered with research and its fantastic results. Many medical researchers try to test hypotheses that are unreasonable, and then draw conclusions unjustified by the methods. The general public only hears that a research was conducted and the positive or negative results as supported by the media. How scientifically and ethically it was conducted is hardly a concern. Because few people are capable of analyzing the published research critically, and evaluating its methodology and procedure, every research is considered equally valid and true. Most researches are prompted by interest groups and lobbyists, and lavishly funded by such interest groups. There is good research and bad research. Bad research takes place more in the field of emotionally loaded and contentious issues like drug abuse, sexuality, birth control, nutrition, management of mental illness, alternative treatments, and so forth. These researches look very scientific by their use of technical jargon, graphs, tables, etc.

However, there are many subjective factors that enter into any research, so much so, that pure objectivity is unlikely. The beliefs and expectations of the researchers, as well as the subject's conscious and unconscious impacts, cannot be overlooked. The mind plays a subtle role that is not measurable by scientific methods. Science that denies the immaterial mind and spirit, I doubt, can produce reliable scientific evidence regarding the complex human organisms on health and healing issues. Medical scientists, who are willing to work from a sound definition of health and healing, and explore new models of reality, will be able to design good research to promote authentic health and healing.

If this book has helped you to think outside of the box of traditional medicine, I am content. The way of looking at health and disease from a different perspective can empower you to choose health. You do not need to be a medical specialist to take care of your health.

Endnotes

Introduction

[1] For a discussion of concise, yet, comprehensive journey that recounts our past and present state of collective knowledge in the diverse fields of biology, medicine, and information technology, see Ray Kurzwell, Terry Grossman, *Fantastic Journey* (Rodalestore USA: Rodale Inc., 2004).

[2] Dean Edell, *Eat, Drink, & Be Merry* (New York: Harper Collins Publishers, 1999), 9.

[3] See Gary Null, *Get Healthy Now* (New York: Seven Stories Press, 2001).

[4] Edward Creagan, *How Not To Be My Patient* (Deerfield Beach, Florida: Health Communications Inc., 2003), 15.

Chapter 1

[1] For an excellent discussion of Health as Wholeness: Wholeness as Perfection, Holiness and Balancing see Andrew Weil, *Health and Healing* (New York: Houghton Mifflin Company), *41-66.*

[2] See Jeff Levin, *God Faith and Health* (John Wiley and Sons, Inc., New York: 2001). Presents a theosomatic model with compelling scientific evidence. His

perspective presents obvious challenge for those stuck in the body or body-mind era of medicine. P. 206.

[3] Weil, Ibid, 92.

[4] Aldous Huxley, *The Perennial Philosophy* (New York: Harper and Row, 1944), 68.

[5] Morton Kelsey, *Christopsychology* (New York: Cross Road Publishing, 1968).

[6] Robert Assagioli, *Psychosynthesis: A Manual of Principles and Techniques.* (New York: Penguin Books, 1976), 61.

[7] Mathew Maniampra, *Wholistic Growth: 100% Life* (Bangalore: Dharmaram Publications, 1997).

[8] Quoted in Caroline Myss and Norman Shealy, *The Creation of Health* (New York: Three River Press, 1993), 11.

[9] Larry Dossey, *Healing Words* (San Francisco: Harper Collins Publishers, 1993). Restores the spiritual art of healing to the science of medicine. The book is a rare one of its kind that challenges outdated medical wisdom.

[10] Weil, Ibid, 36.

[11] See Lao-tzu, *The Way of Life* translated by Witter Bynner, (New York: Capricorn Books, 1962).

Chapter 2

[1] The hologram is produced by a technology that captures and displays an image through the use of lasers. In a hologram, the image of an object is created on a photographic plate by using two separate laser beams that hit the object from different angles. The photography thus produced can be used to recreate the image in three-dimension so that the viewer may move around it and observe it from many angles. This method gives more information about an object than a conventional photograph. The information about the whole is distributed throughout the photograph. Holographic metaphor implies that each piece contains the essence of the whole.

[2] Paul S. Muller, MD; David J. Plevak, MD; and Teresa A. Rummans, MD. "Religious Involvement, Spirituality and Medicine: Implications for Clinical Practice." *Mayo Clinic Proc.* 2001; 76: 1235-1236.

[3] Eric Berne, *Games People Play* (New York: Grove Press, 1964).

[4] Rick Warren's *Purpose Driven Life,* is a modern classic for religious people. He is absolutely brilliant in explaining the real purpose of life on earth and stating profound truths in simple ways. It is a guide to re-script one's life to avoid spiritual stress and its subsequent problems in the over-all health.

[5] Caroline Myss, Norman Shealy, *The Creation of Health* (New York: Three River Press, 1993), 54.

[6] Kelsey, Ibid, 26.

[7] Dale A. Matthews, *The Faith Factor,* (New York: Penguin Books, 1998), 280.

[8] Eugene Taylor, *A Psychology of Spiritual Healing* (West Chester, Pennsylvania: Chrysalis Books, 1999), 26.

[9] Viktor Frankl, *Man's Search for Meaning: An Introduction to Logotherapy* (Boston: Beacon Press, 1963).

[10] Andrew Weil, *Health and Healing* (New York: Houghton Mifflin Company, 1998), 103.

[11] George Vithoulkas, *The Science of Homeopathy* (New York; Grove Press, 1980), 40.

Chapter 3

[1] Rudolph Ballentine presents a masterpiece of sensible healing in the book, *Radical Healing.* One will come across a wonderful blend of the world's most dynamic healing methods. (New York: Harmony Books, 1999).

[2] Guido Manjo, *The Healing Hand: Man and Wound in the Ancient World.* (Cambridge, Mass: Harvard University Press, 1975), 46-48.

[3] Andrew Weil. *8 Weeks to Optimum Health.* (New York: Alfred A. Knopf, 1998) 2-21.

[4] See George Vithoulkas, *The Science of Homeopathy*, for a treatise on the integration of homeopathic and Allopathic principles with an emphasis on the individual as an integrated system. (Grove Press: New York, 1980).

[5] See Ballentine, Ibid, 118.

[6] See Virginia Livingston, MD "Some Cultural, Immunological and Biochemical properties of Progenitor Cryptocides." *Trans NY Academy of Science* 36 (1974), 569-82. Also see Thomas McPherson Brown, MD, "The Road Back" (1988), updated and republished as "The Arthritis Breakthrough" (New York: M. Evans and Co., 1993).

[7] Homeopathic remedies and its different potencies represent different energetic patterns that can correct the energy derangement and the subsequent symptoms.

[8] Quoted in Mark Hyman and Mark Liponis, *Ultra Prevention* (New York: Scribner, 2004), 53.

[9] M. Scott Peck, MD, *The Road Less Traveled* (New York: Touchstone Book, 1979), 19.

[10] Jim Fotin, *The Owners Manual No One Gave You* (New York: PMU Publications 1999), 12.

[11] Helmut Schmidt, "Superposition of Pk effects by Man and Dog", *Research in Parapsychology*, 1983, edited by R. White and R. Broughton (Metuchen, NJ. Scarecrow Press, 1984) 90-98. See also Dean Radin and Roger Nelson, "Consciousness Related Effects in Random Physical Systems," *Foundations of Physics 19, 1989)*: 1499-1514.

[12] Larry Dossey, *Healing Words* (New York: Harper Collins, 1993), 121-123.

[13] Iatrogenic illness is a condition caused by medical personnel in treatment, diagnostic procedures, or being exposed to the environment of a health care facility.

[14] Edward E. Shook, *Elementary Treatise in Herbology* (New York: Enos Publishing Co., 1993), 11.

[15] Weil, Ibid, 105.

[16] George Vithoulkas, *The Science of Homeopathy* (New York: Grove Press, 1980), 6.

[17] Vithoulkas, Ibid, 43.

[18] For a general evaluation of surgical treatments for coronary artery disease, see Eugene Braunwald, *Heart Disease: A Textbook of Cardiovascular Medicine* (Philadelphia: W.B. Saunders, 1980), 418.

Chapter 4

[1] T. P. Archer and C. V. Leier. "Placebo Treatment in Congestive Heart Failure." *Cardiology* 81 (1982), 125-33.

[2] Herbert Benson MD, leader of mind/body medicine, shows us that belief can heal us not only spiritually but physically as well. His book *Timeless Healing* is a gold mine of information about integrative medicine. (New York: Scribner, 1996), 37.

[3] E. G. Dimond, C. F. Kittle, and J. E. Crockett, Comparison of Internal Mammary Litigation and Sham Operation for Angina Pectoris." *American Journal of Cardiology* 5 (1960) 483-486.

[4] John Kehoe, *Mind Power* (Canada: Zoetic Inc., 1997), 113.

[5] Kehoe, Ibid, 5.

6 Andrew Weil, *Health and Healing* (New York: Houghton Mifflin Company), 215.

[7] See H. Benson and M. Epstein, "The placebo Effect of: A neglected Asset in the care of patients," *Journal of the American Medical Association* 232:12 (1975), 1225-27; "The Lie That Heals; The Ethics of Giving Placebos," *Annals of Internal Medicine 97* (1982), 112-18.

[8] Weil, Ibid, 231.

[9] Benson, Ibid, 81.

[10] See Daniel Coleman. *Emotional Intelligence* (New York: Bantam Books, 1995).

Chapter 5

[1] Daniel Coleman, *Working with Emotional Intelligence* (New York: Bantam Books, 1998), 76.

[2] Herbert Benson, *Timeless Healing* (New York: Scribner, 1996), 140.

[3] Mathew Maniampra, *Wholistic Growth: 100% Life* (Bangalore: Dharmaram Publications, 1997), 74.

[4] Rachel Copelan, *How to Hypnotize Yourself and Others.* (Florida: Lifetime Books Inc., 1997), 18.

[5] Benson, Ibid, 133.

[6] Campion, A. A., *Biofeedback Training,* in D. Benner Ed., Baker Encyclopedia of Psychology. (Grand Rapids, Michigan: Baker Book House, 1985).

[7] Copelan, Ibid.

[8] Quoted in Wayne Dyer, *The Wisdom of the Ages* (New York: Harper Collins Publishers, 1998), 179.

[9] Caroline Myss, Norman Shealy, *The Creation of Health,* (New York: Three River Press, 1993), 32.

[10] Dyer, Ibid, 180.

[11] D. B. Larson, S. S. Larson, and J.P. Sweyers, *The Costly Consequences of Divorce* (Rockville, MD; National Institute for Healthcare Research, 1996); Interview with David B. Larson, MD, May 23, 1997.

[12] Myss and Shealy, Ibid, 23.

[13] Rudolph Ballentine, *Radical Healing* (New York: Harmony Books, 1999).

[14] Stephen Arturburn, *Hand Me Down Genes and Second Hand Emotions* (Nashville: Thomas Nelson Publishers, 1992), 26.

Chapter 6

[1] Rene Dubos, *Mirage of Health: Utopias, Progress and Biological Change* (New York: Harper and Brothers, 1959), 110.

[2] Bill Gottlieb (ed.), *New Choices in Natural Healing* (Emmaus, Pennsylvania; Rodale Press Inc., 1995), 9.

[3] Gottlieb, Ibid, 12.

[4] Edward Shook, *Elementary Treatise in Herbology* (Banning, CA. Enos Publishing Co., 1993), 11.

[5] Gottlieb, Ibid, 43.

[6] Gary Null, *Ultimate Anti-Aging Program* (New York: Kensington Publishing Corp., 199), 7.

[7] James F. Balch, Phyllis A. Balch, *Nutritional Healing* (New York: Avery Publishing Group, 1993), 5.

[8] Rudolph Ballentine, *Diet and Nutrition A Holistic Approach, (*Hondsdale, Pa., Himalayan Publishers 1978). A comprehensive textbook of nutrition covering agricultural, biochemical, physiological, psychological and philosophical aspects of nutrition.

[9] Ballentine, *Radical Healing* (New York: Harmony Books, 1999), 263.

[10] Elson M. Hass, *The Detox Diet* (Berkeley, CA; Celestial Arts Publishing, 1996), 22.

[11] Hass, Ibid, 114.

Chapter 7

1 Rudolph Ballentine, *Radical Healing* (New York: Harmony Books, 1999), 142.

[2] Samuel Hahnemann, *Organon of the Medical Art,* 6th edition based on a translation by Steven Decker, edited and annotated by Wenda B. O'Reilly (Washington: Birdcage Books, 1979), 19.

[3] Steven B. Kayne, *Homeopathic Pharmacy (*Singapore: Churchill Livingstone, 1977), 86.

[4] George Vithoulkas, *The Science of Homeopathy* (New York: Grove Press, 1980).

[5] Vithoulkas, Ibid, 78.

[6] James Tyler Kent, *Lectures on Homeopathic Philosophy* (California: North Atlantic Books, 1977), 21.

[7] Hahnemann, Ibid, 66.

[8] Hahnemann, Ibid, 61.

[9] Edward Cotter, *Homeopathic Teachings from a Master (*Essex: C. W. Daniel Co. Ltd., 1987), 10.

[10] Jerome D. Frank, *A Comparative Study of Psychotherapy* (Baltimore: Johns Hopkins University Press, 1961), 37.

Chapter 8

[1] Paul S. Muller, David J. Plevak, Teresa A. Rummans. Review: Religious Involvement, Spirituality, and Medicine Implications for Clinical Practice. Mayo Foundation for Medical Education and Research. Mayo Clinic Proc. (2001); 76: 1225-1235.

[2] W. A. Oleckno and M. J. Blacconiere, "Relationship of Religiosity to Wellness and Other Health-Related Behaviors and Outcomes" *Psychological Reports* (1991) 819-26.

[3] D. M. Johnson, J. S. Williams and D. G. Bromley, "Religion, Health and Healing; Findings from a Southern City," *Sociological Analysis 46* (1986), 66-73.

[4] Herbert Benson, *Timeless Healing* (New York: Scribner, 1996), 168.

[5] Mayo Clinic Proc, Ibid, 1225-1227.

[6] Koenig H G, Chen H J, Blazer D G, et al., "Religious coping and depression among elderly, hospitalized, medically ill men" *American Journal of Psychiatry* (1992) 149; 1693-1700.

[7] Kenneth Caine and Brian Kaufman, *Prayer Faith and Healing* (Pennsylvania: Rodale Press, Inc., 1999).

[8] R.C. Ness and R.M. Winthrop, "The Emotional Impact of Fundamentalist Religious Participation: an Empirical Study of Intragroup Variation," *American Journal of Orthopsychiatry* 50, No. 2 (1980), 302-14.

9 Dale A. Matthews, *The Faith Factor* (New York: Penguin Books, 1998), 135.

[10] F. Berkman and S. L. Syme, "Social Networks, Host, Resistance and Mortality," *American Journal of Epidemiology* 19 (1979), 186-204.

[11] Quoted in Matthews, 107.

[12] H. W. Gibbs and J. Acterberg Lawlis. "Spiritual Values and Death Anxiety: Implications for Counseling with Terminal Cancer Patients," *Journal of Counseling Psychology* 25, No. 6 (1978), 563-69.

[13] Matthews, Ibid.

[14] Larry Dossey, *Healing Beyond the Body* (Boston: Shambala, 2001), 242.

[15] Matthews, Ibid, 41.

[16] Gordon W. Allport and J. Michael Ross "Personal Religious Orientation and Prejudice." *Journal of Personality and Social Psychology* 5, No. 2 (1967), 432-443.

[17] Matthews, Ibid, 55.

Chapter 9

[1] Jung quoted in R. Walsh and F. Vaughn, (eds.) *Paths Beyond Ego: The Transpersonal Vision* (Los Angeles: J. P. Tarcher, 1993).

[2] Ted Schwarz, *Healing in the Name of the Lord* (Grand Rapids, Michigan: Zondervan Publishing House, 1993), 117.

[3] William G. Braud, "Consciousness Interactions with Remote Biological Systems: Anomalous Intentionality Effects," *Subtle Energies* (Journal of the International Society for the Study of Subtle Energies and Energy Medicine) 2, No.1: 1-46.

[4] Schwarz, Ibid, 20.

[5] Schwarz, Ibid, 23.

[6] According to the laws of chemistry, there is a limit to the serial dilutions that can be made without losing the original substance altogether. Any potency beyond 24x or 12c has virtually no chance of containing even one molecule of the original substance. In homeopathic practice, it is seen that potencies ranging far beyond this limit, even over 100,000c continue to be effective.

Printed in the United States
52565LVS00005B/202-366

9 781425 917975